The Ultimate Beginner's Guide to Herbalism

Discover 200+ Natural Remedies and Medicinal Herbs to Grow Your Own Medicine, Become Self-Sufficient, and Build Your At-Home Apothecary

The Green Glow

Contents

Freebies For Our Supporters!

We've got a nice beginner recipe book for all of you herbal newbies out there. Just scan the code below to claim yours!

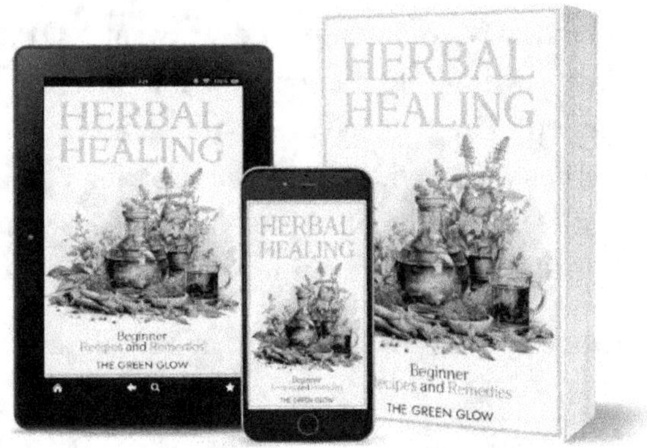

I want my freebie!

Join Our Budding Community!

We have a brand new community and we want **YOU** to help us grow! Are you willing to be one of the first seeds in our Facebook garden? Do you have any questions? Do you want share your herbal world with us and our glowing community? If you answered yes to any of these then, well, what are you waiting for? Just scan the code to join our community!

Join the Facebook group: Herbs, Heart, and Healing

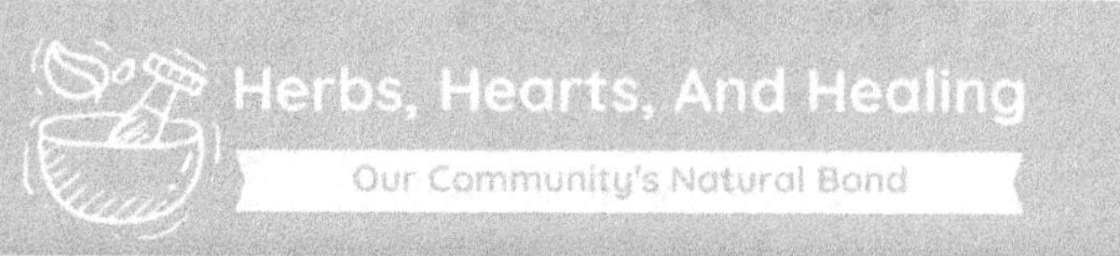

Introduction

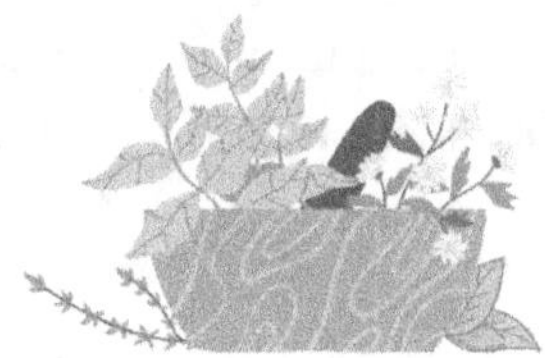

Welcome to the enchanting world of herbalism, where the bounty of nature unfolds its secrets to you if you are curious enough to listen. Herbalism, at its essence, is the art and science of harnessing the healing properties of plants to nourish the body and promote general well-being. It's a timeless practice that spans millennia across cultures and civilizations around the world. It's rooted in the profound connection between humans and the abundant gifts of the Earth.

In this beginner's guide, we invite you to embark on a journey that explores the wisdom of herbs and their remarkable ability to nurture the body, mind, and spirit. Whether you are drawn to the therapeutic qualities of plants, seeking natural alternatives to support health, or simply captivated by the magic of the green world, herbalism offers a gateway to a healthy and harmonious way of living.

—Imagine walking through a fragrant garden surrounded by a kaleidoscope of colors and textures—each plant telling a story of resilience and healing. Herbalism is like communicating with these botanical storytellers, learning from their ancient wisdom, and discovering the treasures they hold within their leaves, flowers, roots, and stems.

As we embark on this herbal journey together, we'll demystify the language of plants, explore the basic principles of herbalism, and empower you with the knowledge to create your own herbal remedies. So, grab a cup of herbal tea, breathe in the earthy aromas, and let's dive into the fascinating world of herbalism—a journey of discovery, connection, and well-being.

Chapter 1

The Roots of Herbalism

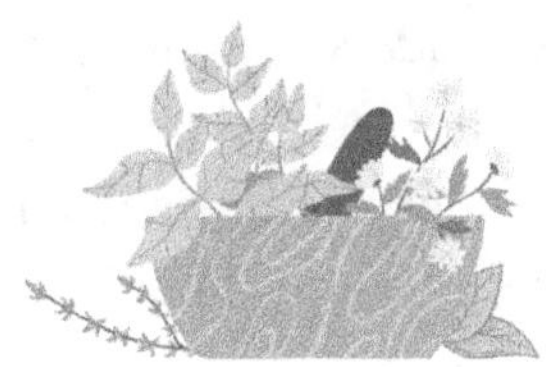

What is Herbalism?

Herbalism, often referred to as herbal medicine or phytotherapy, is a holistic approach to healing and well-being that draws upon the therapeutic properties of plants to promote well-being, prevent illness, and address various health conditions.

Rooted in ancient traditions and evolving through the ages, herbalism encapsulates a deeper understanding of the intricate relationship between humans and the plant kingdom. As people increasingly seek alternative approaches to health, the resurgence of herbalism is a testament to the enduring power of plants in nurturing the body, mind, and spirit.

The Principles of Herbalism

At its core, herbalism operates on the principle that plants contain a myriad of chemical compounds with diverse medicinal properties. These compounds such as alkaloids, flavonoids, and essential oils interact with the human body in intricate ways, thus, influencing physiological functions and supporting the body's natural healing processes.

A Holistic Approach

One of the defining features of herbalism is its holistic perspective. Rather than focusing solely on symptoms or isolated aspects of health, herbalism considers the entire person—mind, body, and spirit. This holistic approach acknowledges the interconnectedness of the body's various systems and emphasizes the importance of addressing the root causes of imbalances.

The Herbalist's Toolbox

Herbalists use an array of plant parts from different species, including leaves, flowers, roots, stems, and seeds, to create remedies. These can take various forms, such as teas, tinctures, salves, poultices, and capsules. Choosing a method of preparing herbal remedies often depends on the properties of the plant and the desired therapeutic effect.

Traditional Wisdom and Cultural Variations

Herbalism has been deeply ingrained in the traditions of diverse cultures worldwide. Each culture has its own herbal knowledge passed down through generations often reflecting the unique plants native to the region. Traditional Chinese medicine (TCM), Ayurveda, Native American herbalism, European herbal traditions, and many other lesser-known herbal remedies from all around the world contribute to the rich tapestry of our global herbal heritage.

Energetics and Constitutional Approaches

Herbalism sometimes employs the concept of energetics where plants are classified based on their inherent qualities—hot, cold, damp, dry, etc. This classification could help to tailor remedies to someone's constitution and the specific imbalances they may be experiencing. It's a highly personalized approach that takes the uniqueness of each person's constitution into account.

Scientific Inquiry and Modern Herbalism

While deeply rooted in tradition, herbalism is not stagnant. Modern herbalists often integrate up-to-date scientific research and evidence-based practices into their approach. This marriage of traditional wisdom and contemporary understanding enhances the credibility of herbalism in a world that demands evidence-driven healthcare.

Preventive Care and Wellness Promotion

Herbalism is not solely about treating illnesses; it emphasizes preventive care and the promotion of overall wellness. Many herbs possess adaptogenic qualities, helping the body adapt to stressors and maintain balance. This preventive aspect aligns with the philosophy of supporting the body's innate healing capacities, aids in bolstering the immune system, and promotes physical and mental well-being.

Cultural, Spiritual, and Sustainable Aspects

Beyond the purely medicinal, herbalism often carries cultural and spiritual significance. Plants may be used in rituals, ceremonies, or as symbols of cultural identity. Additionally, herbalism emphasizes sustainable practices, hence, encouraging ethical harvesting, cultivation, and conservation of plant species to ensure the continued availability of medicinal plants, especially when they are a protected species or from sensitive ecosystems.

A Brief History of Herbalism

Long before the advent of modern medicine and pharmaceuticals, our ancestors turned to the natural world for remedies and healing. The ancient civilizations that dotted the globe were pioneers in the art of herbalism cultivating an intimate relationship with the plants that surrounded them. This profound connection with nature laid the foundation for the rich variety of herbal traditions we know and practice today.

Mesopotamia and Sumeria: The Cradle of Herbal Knowledge

In ancient Mesopotamia and Sumeria, herbalism was intricately woven into daily life. Medical cuneiform tablets—some dating back to 3000 B.C.E.—reveal a sophisticated understanding of medicinal plants. The Sumerians—with their advanced knowledge of agriculture and botany—cultivated and traded various herbs. Herbal wisdom was interwoven with religious and magical beliefs, therefore, showcasing the holistic nature of healing.

Mesopotamian contributions laid the groundwork for herbal traditions, subsequently influencing the evolving practices that would shape the history of medicine in the ancient world.

China: The Preservers of Early Herbalism

Herbalism in China traces back over 2,500 years rooted in ancient texts like the Huangdi Neijing. The famous *Pen-Ts'ao Ching* of ancient China, often considered the earliest comprehensive herbal text, showcased the Chinese civilization's profound respect for the healing power of plants. Influenced by Daoist and Confucian philosophies, Chinese herbalists explored the intricate balance of Yin and Yang, the Five Elements, and Qi. Key figures like Li Shizhen's *Compendium of Materia Medica* enriched herbal knowledge.

Despite challenges during the 20th century, China's commitment to traditional medicine led to a revival. Today, TCM integrates herbal remedies, acupuncture, and holistic principles into mainstream healthcare, subsequently contributing to and influencing global wellness practices.

Ancient Egypt: Botanical Elixirs and Beyond

The ancient Egyptians known for their advanced medical practices were early herbalists. More than 40 papyrus scrolls dating back to 1800 B.C.E. contain extensive lists of herbal remedies and uses in medicine, showcasing their deep knowledge of plants like aloe, garlic, and myrrh. The Ebers papyrus from 1550 B.C.E. lists more than 700 formulas for medicinal herbal remedies. Plants were used not just for medicinal purposes but they played a vital role in religious ceremonies and daily rituals, thus, emphasizing the holistic nature of herbalism in Egyptian culture.

Greek Wisdom and the Birth of Western Herbalism

Ancient Greece may be more well known as the cradle of philosophy and science, but the Greeks also contributed significantly to herbalism. An oral history of herbal uses exists in the Homeric hymns and epics from the 8th century B.C.E. Later, from the 5th and 4th centuries B.C.E., the works of Hippocrates and Theophrastus became pillars of herbal knowledge.

Hippocrates, often hailed as the "Father of Medicine," emphasized the importance of treating the whole person, thus, laying the groundwork for holistic herbal practices. Theophrastus—a student of Aristotle—meticulously studied and often discussed plants, their uses, methods of harvest, as well as the effects these plants have on humans and animals. He essentially began the science of botany by classifying the plants in the botanical gardens of Athens in his *Historia Plantarum,* or *Theophrastus Book*—a botanical taxonomy that influenced herbalism for centuries.

Ayurveda in Ancient India: Harmony and Balance

In ancient India, the wisdom of herbalism found expression in Ayurveda—a holistic system of medicine that sought balance in mind, body, and spirit. Dating back over 5,000 years in India, Ayurveda is a system of herbalism rooted in ancient medical texts like the Charaka Samhita and Sushruta Samhita. Developed by sages, Ayurveda harmonizes the body, mind, and spirit through personalized treatments, emphasizing the balance of body energies called doshas.

Herbal remedies play a pivotal role with extensive knowledge passed down through generations. Ayurveda's holistic approach extends beyond physical health, thereafter embracing mental and spiritual well-being. Today, Ayurveda persists as a dynamic force influencing global wellness practices and affirming its enduring relevance in the realm of herbal medicine.

Indigenous Herbalism: A Living Tradition

While the ancient civilizations of Mesopotamia, Egypt, Greece, and India left a lasting legacy, it is important to acknowledge the enduring herbal traditions of indigenous cultures worldwide. Native American, African, Australian Aboriginal, and other indigenous societies have cultivated an intimate knowledge of their local plants, using them for nourishment, healing, spiritual, and cultural practices.

The roots of herbalism run deep in the annals of human history. Ancient civilizations, with their reverence for nature and keen observation, paved the way for the herbal traditions we cherish today.

The Modern Resurgence of Herbalism: Nurturing Nature's Renaissance

In recent decades, there has been a remarkable resurgence of interest in herbalism, marking a return to nature's remedies and a rediscovery of traditional healing practices. Herbalism is characterized by a growing awareness of the therapeutic potential of plants, a desire for more natural approaches to healthcare, and an appreciation for the holistic wisdom that herbalism offers. Let us delve into the factors contributing to the modern resurgence of herbalism:

Shift Towards Holistic Wellness

As people seek holistic approaches to well-being, herbalism has emerged as a comprehensive and integrative system. Modern lifestyles—often marked by stress, environmental pollutants, and detached from nature—have led people to explore holistic alternatives that address physical, mental, and emotional aspects of their health. Herbalism, with its emphasis on treating the whole person, aligns seamlessly with this shift towards holistic wellness.

Backlash Against Synthetic Pharmaceuticals

The side effects and environmental impact associated with synthetic pharmaceuticals have spurred a quest for gentler alternatives. Many people are turning to herbal remedies as a safer, more sustainable option. The desire for treatments with fewer adverse effects has led to a reevaluation of the efficacy of herbal preparations, hence, contributing to the renewed popularity of herbalism.

Access to Information

The digital age has democratized information, thus, allowing people to access a wealth of knowledge about herbalism. Blogs, online forums, social media, and educational platforms provide a space for enthusiasts to share experiences, recipes, and information about herbal practices. This easy access to information has empowered people to experiment with herbal remedies and integrate them into their daily lives.

Cultural and Environmental Consciousness

A growing awareness of the environmental impact of modern lifestyles has prompted a reevaluation of consumption patterns including healthcare choices. Herbalism with its emphasis on sustainable and locally sourced remedies aligns with the principles of environmental consciousness. The desire to reconnect with cultural roots and traditional practices has fueled an interest in herbalism as a way to tap into ancestral knowledge.

Scientific Validation of Traditional Knowledge

Traditional herbal knowledge passed down through generations is gaining recognition in scientific circles. Researchers are increasingly exploring the therapeutic properties of plants, validating the efficacy of traditional remedies. This intersection of traditional wisdom and scientific inquiry has contributed to the credibility of herbalism in the eyes of a modern, evidence-driven audience.

Rise of Herbal Education and Certification

Educational programs and certifications in herbalism have proliferated, offering structured learning opportunities for those interested in mastering the art. This formalization of herbal education has not only elevated the status of herbalism but has also created a community of trained practitioners who contribute to the dissemination of herbal knowledge.

The modern resurgence of herbalism is driven by a convergence of factors ranging from a desire for holistic wellness to a reevaluation of conventional healthcare practices. As herbalism continues to weave itself into the fabric of contemporary health and lifestyle choices, it's both a return to ancient wisdom and an innovative response to the evolving needs of a health-conscious and nature-loving society.

Cultural Significance of Herbs Across Various Civilizations

The use of herbs holds profound cultural significance across diverse societies, shaping traditions, spirituality, and daily practices. Let us take a look at how different cultures incorporate herbs into their customs, rituals, and daily lives:

Native American Traditions

In Native American cultures, herbs play a central role in spiritual practices and healing ceremonies. Sage, cedar, sweetgrass, and tobacco are often used in smudging rituals to cleanse and purify spaces. Each herb holds specific symbolic meanings and is believed to connect people with the spirit world, ancestors, and the natural elements.

Chinese Herbalism

TCM has a rich tradition of herbalism dating back thousands of years. Herbs integral to TCM formulations like ginseng, astragalus, and licorice root are believed to restore balance in the body's vital energy called Qi. Chinese herbalism addresses physical ailments while also considering the energetic qualities of herbs and their impact on the body's meridian system.

Ayurvedic Healing

Ayurveda relies heavily on herbal remedies. Herbs like turmeric, ashwagandha, and neem have various roles in promoting balance among the three doshas—Vata, Pitta, and Kapha. Ayurvedic practice encompasses mental, emotional, and spiritual well-being.

European Herbal Traditions

Herbalism has deep roots in European cultures where traditional remedies have been passed down through generations. Herbs like chamomile, lavender, and thyme are used for their calming properties and culinary applications. European folklore is rich with herbal symbolism, and many herbs were believed to possess protective qualities against supernatural forces.

African Herbalism

Across the vast and diverse continent of Africa, various ethnic groups have distinct herbal traditions. The San and the Khoikoi from southern Africa have a vast knowledge of the native desert flora that has been passed down generations for centuries. Herbs are used not only for medicinal purposes but also in rituals, ceremonies, and rites of passage. In some cultures, the knowledge of herbal remedies is guarded by herbalists who strictly pass it down within their families.

Herbs in Middle Eastern Cultures

Middle Eastern cultures have a long history of herbal use for both culinary and medicinal purposes. Herbs like mint, thyme, and coriander are staples in Middle Eastern cuisine. Additionally, traditional healing practices influenced by Islamic medicine incorporate herbs to address a range of health issues.

Latin American Herbalism

Indigenous cultures in Latin America have a deep connection to the rich biodiversity of the region. Herbs like coca, aloe vera, and guayusa have been used for centuries for their culinary and medicinal properties. The cultural significance extends to spiritual ceremonies where herbs are often used to invoke protection, introspection, and healing.

Herbs in Neopaganism and Wicca

In neo-paganism and Wiccan traditions, herbs hold symbolic and magical significance. Wiccans, druids, herbalists, and practitioners of various magical arts incorporate herbs into spells, potions, and rituals. Each herb is believed to carry specific energies aligning with intentions for healing, protection, or spiritual enhancement.

Japanese Kampo Medicine

Japan has its own herbal tradition known as Kampo which blends Chinese herbal principles with traditional Japanese practices. Herbs like ginger, licorice, and cinnamon are used in Kampo formulations to address imbalances and promote overall health.

Herbs in Jewish and Islamic Traditions

Both Jewish and Islamic cultures have historical connections to herbalism. In Jewish traditions, herbs like hyssop and myrtle are used in rituals, while Islamic medicine incorporates various herbs like black seed and dates for their therapeutic properties.

Exploring the Benefits and Reasons to Embrace Herbalism

The benefits and reasons to explore herbalism are diverse and compelling. From its holistic approach to well-being to its cultural connections, personalized care, and sustainability, herbalism offers a multifaceted journey toward health that will resonate with you if you're seeking a natural, empowering, and harmonious path to well-being. Let us take a look at some of the numerous benefits and compelling reasons to delve into the world of herbalism:

Natural Healing and Holistic Well-Being

Herbalism emphasizes natural healing, focusing on the body's innate ability to restore balance. The holistic approach of herbalism addresses not only physical symptoms but also considers the interconnectedness of mental, emotional, and spiritual well-being. By treating the whole person, herbal remedies aim to support overall health and harmony.

Gentle and Fewer Side Effects

Many herbal remedies are known for their gentle nature and minimal side effects compared to some synthetic pharmaceuticals. This makes herbalism an attractive option, especially for people who may have allergies or sensitivities to conventional medications or are seeking alternatives with fewer adverse effects.

Cultural and Traditional Connection

Exploring herbalism allows you to connect with cultural traditions and ancestral wisdom. Many cultures worldwide have deep-rooted herbal practices. Learning about and practicing herbalism provides an opportunity to rediscover and honor this cultural heritage, thereby fostering a sense of connection to the past.

Empowerment Through Self-Care

Herbalism encourages a proactive approach to health and empowers you to take an active role in your well-being. Learning about herbs and their uses enables you to create your own remedies, therefore, making you more self-sufficient and in control over your own health and well-being.

Preventive Health and Immune Support

Herbal remedies often have preventive qualities, supporting the body's immune system and helping to ward off illness. Adaptogenic herbs, for example, can assist the body in adapting to stressors, thus, promoting resilience and overall health. This preventive aspect aligns with the philosophy of maintaining balance before imbalances manifest as illness.

Personalized and Individualized Care

Herbalism allows for personalized and individualized care as herbalists often consider a person's unique constitution, lifestyle, and specific health concerns when crafting remedies. This tailored approach acknowledges that each person may respond differently to herbs and emphasizes the importance of personalized care.

Accessible and Sustainable

As a result of our global society, herbs from all around the world are often readily available, and many can be cultivated or foraged locally. This accessibility makes herbalism an inclusive and sustainable option for promoting health.

The focus on sustainable harvesting and cultivation aligns with eco-conscious values, contributing to the preservation of plant species and ecosystems.

Versatility in Applications

Herbalism offers a wide range of applications, from teas and tinctures to salves, poultices, capsules, and even culinary uses. The versatility of herbs allows you to incorporate them into various aspects of daily life making herbal remedies easy to integrate into existing routines.

Mind-Body Connection and Emotional Wellness

Herbalism recognizes the intimate connection between the mind and body. Many herbs have properties that influence emotional well-being that help alleviate stress, anxiety, and other emotional imbalances. This mind-body approach contributes to the holistic healing that herbalism offers.

Cultivation of Nature Connection

Herbalism enables you to connect with nature on a deeper level. Whether through cultivating a medicinal herb garden, foraging for wild plants, or simply learning about the properties of plants you can find locally, herbalism encourages you to appreciate and learn from the natural world around you.

Distinguishing Herbalism, Homeopathy, and Conventional Medicine

Herbalism, homeopathy, and conventional medicine are distinct approaches to healthcare each with its own philosophy, principles, and methodologies. Understanding the differences between them is essential when seeking alternative avenues of treatment.

Herbalism

Philosophy

Holistic approach: Herbalism takes a holistic approach to health considering the interconnectedness of the body, mind, and spirit. It aims to address the root causes of imbalances rather than merely alleviating symptoms.

Nature-based: Herbalism relies on the therapeutic properties of plants. It acknowledges the innate healing wisdom of nature and emphasizes the use of plant preparations to support well-being.

Methodology

Herb selection: Herbalists choose plants based on their traditional uses, properties, and energetics. They may use leaves, flowers, roots, and other plant parts to create remedies such as teas, tinctures, salves, and poultices.

Personalized care: Herbalists often consider a person's constitution, lifestyle, and specific health concerns when crafting remedies while recognizing that people may respond differently to herbal remedies.

Cultural and Historical Context

Herbalism has a rich history across diverse cultures with practices deeply rooted in traditional knowledge passed down through generations. Cultural and regional herbal traditions contribute to the diversity of herbal practices.

Homeopathy

Philosophy

Law of similarity: Homeopathy operates on the belief that "like cures like," wherein a substance which causes symptoms in an otherwise healthy person can be diluted and used to alleviate similar symptoms in an unwell person suffering those same symptoms.

Energy medicine: Homeopathy posits that diluting and shaking a substance in a specific manner enhances its healing energy while minimizing toxicity.

Methodology

High dilution: Homeopathic remedies are highly diluted substances often to the point where the original substance may not be detectable. This extreme dilution is believed to enhance the remedy's healing properties.

Individualized treatment: Homeopathic practitioners conduct detailed interviews to understand a person's physical, emotional, and mental symptoms. Remedies are then prescribed based on the totality of symptoms.

Cultural and Historical Context

Homeopathy was founded in the late 18th century by the German physician Samuel Hahnemann. It has since evolved and gained popularity as an alternative therapeutic system.

Conventional Medicine

Philosophy

Evidence-based: Conventional medicine, also known as allopathic or Western medicine, is evidence-based and relies on scientific research to create medicines and to establish the safety and efficacy of treatments.

Symptom management: The primary focus is on curing ailments and managing symptoms using medications, surgery, and other interventions.

Methodology

Pharmaceutical interventions: Conventional medicine frequently employs pharmaceutical drugs, surgeries, and other technological interventions to treat diseases and alleviate symptoms.

Specialization: Conventional medicine is highly specialized with practitioners often focusing on specific organ systems or diseases.

Cultural and Historical Context

Conventional medicine has its roots in the scientific revolution and is driven by advancements in medical research, technology, and pharmacology. It has evolved over time, testing the efficacy of old as well as new treatments and incorporating what works into conventional medical practices.

Key Differences	Herbalism	Homeopathy	Conventional Medicine
Source of therapeutic Agents	Relies on the therapeutic properties of whole plants.	Utilizes highly diluted substances often originating from plants, minerals, or animals.	Primarily employs synthetic pharmaceuticals, surgical procedures, and technological interventions.
Approach to holism	Embraces a holistic approach considering the whole person and addressing root causes.	Aims for holistic treatment by considering physical, emotional, and mental symptoms.	Tends to focus on specific symptoms or diseases often with specialized interventions.
Treatment philosophy	Often emphasizes preventive care, balance, and the body's natural healing abilities.	Grounded in the principle of "like cures like" and the enhancement of vital energy.	Primarily focuses on managing symptoms and treating diseases using scientifically validated methods.

While herbalism, homeopathy, and conventional medicine each offer distinct approaches to healthcare, they can also complement each other. The choice between them often depends on your preferences, cultural background, and your specific health needs. It's crucial to make informed decisions, considering the strengths and limitations of each approach, and, consulting healthcare professionals for guidance when necessary.

Chapter 2

Safety and Ethical Considerations

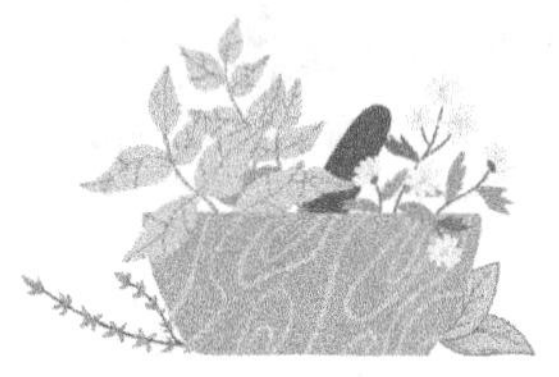

Plant Identification

Importance of Plant Identification

Plant identification is a fundamental skill in various fields encompassing botany, ecology, agriculture, horticulture, herbalism, and conservation. Understanding and distinguishing different plant species are crucial for several reasons:

Biodiversity Conservation

Identifying plant species is essential for monitoring and conserving biodiversity. It allows scientists and conservationists to track the health and distribution of plant populations, aiding in the preservation of ecosystems.

Ecological Studies

Plant identification is fundamental in ecological research. It helps researchers understand the interactions between plant species, their role in the ecosystem, and how environmental changes may impact plant communities.

Agriculture and Horticulture

Farmers and gardeners need to identify plants to optimize cultivation practices. Proper identification ensures the use of appropriate fertilizers, pesticides, and care practices for specific crops or ornamental plants.

Herbalism and Traditional Medicine

Herbalists rely on plant identification to select the right herbs for medicinal purposes. Knowing the distinct features of plants helps ensure the correct identification and use of therapeutic species.

Foraging and Wild Crafting

People who forage for wild edibles or practice wild crafting for herbal remedies must accurately identify plants to ensure safety and to harvest sustainably.

Land Management

In forestry and land management, plant identification is crucial for assessing vegetation health, managing invasive species, and making informed decisions about land use.

Tools for Plant Identification

Several tools are available to aid in plant identification ranging from traditional field guides to modern technology:

Field Guides

- **Books**: Traditional field guides provide detailed descriptions, illustrations, and photographs of plant species. These guides are organized by plant families, making them valuable for in-depth study.
- **Online resources**: Many field guides are available in digital formats allowing users to access information through websites or mobile apps. Websites like

iNaturalist, PlantSnap, and various regional flora databases offer extensive plant identification resources.

Botanical Keys

- **Printed keys**: Botanical keys are dichotomous guides that use a series of paired choices to lead users to the correct identification. They often require a basic understanding of botanical terms.
- **Digital keys**: Some botanical keys are available as interactive digital tools, allowing users to answer questions about a plant's characteristics to narrow down the identification.

Smartphone Apps

Apps like PlantNet, Seek by iNaturalist, and PictureThis utilize image recognition technology to identify plants based on photographs. Users can take pictures of leaves, flowers, or the whole plant for identification.

Online Databases and Websites

- **Flora databases**: Online databases such as USDA Plants Database, Flora of North America, and The Plant List provide comprehensive information about plant species, including distribution, taxonomy, and images.
- **Community platforms**: Websites like iNaturalist and eBird allow users to contribute observations and seek identification help from a community of experts and enthusiasts.

Botanical Gardens and Arboreta

Visiting botanical gardens and arboreta provides an opportunity to learn from curated plant collections. Many institutions offer guided tours or educational programs on plant identification.

Microscopy and Laboratory Techniques

- **Botanical microscopy**: In-depth plant identification may involve microscopic examination of plant parts such as leaves, stems, or seeds using botanical microscopes.
- **Chemical tests**: Some identification may require chemical tests to detect specific compounds or features, especially in herbalism or plant taxonomy.

Accurate plant identification often requires a combination of these tools; ongoing learning and practice significantly enhance proficiency. It's essential to approach plant identification with curiosity, attention to detail, and a commitment to ethical foraging and conservation practices.

Recognizing "Look-Alike Plants" and Their Dangers

Foraging for wild edibles or engaging in plant-related activities requires a keen understanding of plant identification to ensure safety. "Look-alike plants" are species that resemble each other often sharing similar features such as leaves, flowers, or growth habits. However, while some look-alikes are harmless, others may pose risks including toxicity or allergenic properties. Understanding how to differentiate between similar-looking plants is crucial for safe foraging and outdoor activities. Here's how to recognize look-alike plants and the potential dangers associated with misidentification:

Understanding Look-Alike Plants

Similarities

- **Leaves**: Look-alike plants often have similar leaf shapes, sizes, and arrangements.
- **Flowers**: Similarities in flower color, shape, and arrangement may contribute to confusion.
- **Habitat**: Plants with shared ecological niches or habitats may resemble each other.

Common Look-Alikes

- **Wild carrot vs. poison hemlock**: Both belong to the carrot family (*Apiaceae*) and their leaves and flowers share similarities. However, poison hemlock is highly toxic.
- **Chicory vs. wild lettuce**: The blue flowers of chicory can resemble wild lettuce, but the latter can have milky sap and is often bitter-tasting.
- **Edible berries vs. poisonous berries**: Some edible berries have toxic look-alikes such as the toxic berries of the deadly nightshade plant resembling those of certain edible berries.

The Dangers of Misidentification

Toxicity

- **Poisonous plants**: Misidentifying toxic plants can lead to severe poisoning, affecting the digestive, nervous, or respiratory systems.
- **Allergic reactions**: Some look-alike plants may cause allergic reactions, ranging from mild irritation to severe responses.

Mimicry and Camouflage

Some toxic plants closely resemble edible varieties. Mistaking a toxic species for an edible one can have life-threatening consequences.

Misidentification in Herbalism

Look-alike plants may be mistaken for beneficial medicinal herbs leading to improper use and potential health risks.

Tips for Safe Identification

Field Guides and Resources

- **Use reliable guides**: Carry reputable field guides or use trustworthy online resources to cross-reference plant features.
- **Digital apps**: Utilize plant identification apps that use image recognition technology. However, exercise caution and confirm identifications with multiple sources.

Pay Attention to Details

- **Botanical features**: Observe details such as leaf arrangement, shape, color, and texture, as well as flower structure.
- **Habitat and location**: Consider the plant's habitat, geographic location, and the season, as these factors can aid in accurate identification.

Consult Experts

- **Community forums**: Seek guidance from experienced foragers, herbalists, or botanists on community platforms like iNaturalist or local foraging groups.
- **Local botanical gardens**: Attend workshops or events organized by botanical gardens or nature centers to learn from experts.

Err on the Side of Caution

- **When in doubt, leave it out**: If you're uncertain about a plant's identity, it's safer to refrain from consuming or using it.
- **Progress gradually**: As a forager or herbalist, gradually expand your knowledge and confidence over time rather than attempting to identify numerous species all at once.

Documenting and Recording

Keep detailed notes and take clear photographs of the plants you encounter. Keeping records like these can simplify identification in the future.

Continuous Learning and Awareness

Stay Updated

- **Seasonal variations**: Plants may exhibit different characteristics during various seasons. Be aware of these changes.
- **New discoveries**: Stay informed about new discoveries or taxonomic changes within plant species.

Local Variations

Some plant species may have regional variations. Be aware of local nuances in plant identification.

The Dangers of Contamination, Adulteration, and Potential Allergens

While herbalism offers a holistic approach to health and well-being, it's essential to be aware of potential dangers associated with the use of herbal remedies. Three significant concerns in the world of herbalism are contamination, adulteration, and the presence of potential allergens.

Contamination

Contamination in herbalism refers to the unintended presence of harmful substances such as pesticides, heavy metals, or microbial pathogens, in herbal products.

Causes

- **Pesticides and herbicides**: Residual pesticides from cultivation practices can contaminate herbs.
- **Heavy metals**: Plants grown in contaminated soil may absorb heavy metals like lead, mercury, or cadmium.
- **Microbial pathogens**: Improper handling, storage, or processing of herbs can introduce microbial contaminants.

Potential Dangers

- **Toxicity**: Contaminants may pose health risks, leading to toxicity and adverse effects.

- **Microbial infections**: Contaminated herbs may harbor bacteria, fungi, or other pathogens that can cause infections.

Preventive Measures

- **Organic and sustainable practices**: Choose herbs grown using organic and sustainable cultivation practices to minimize pesticide contamination.
- **Testing and quality assurance**: Purchase herbs from reputable suppliers who conduct rigorous testing for contaminants.
- **Good agricultural and collection practices (GACP)**: Adhering to GACP guidelines ensures proper cultivation and harvesting practices to reduce contamination risks. Adhering to GACP guidelines ensures proper cultivation and harvesting practices to reduce contamination risks.

Adulteration

Adulteration involves the intentional addition of substances to herbal products with the aim of increasing weight, volume, potency, or mimicking the appearance of a higher-quality product.

Causes

- **Economic motives**: Adulteration may be driven by economic incentives to increase profit margins.
- **Supply chain complexity**: As herbs pass through various stages of the supply chain, opportunities for adulteration increase.

Potential Dangers

- **Reduced efficacy**: Adulterated products may lack the expected therapeutic benefits.
- **Safety concerns**: The addition of unknown substances may introduce allergens or toxic compounds.

Preventive Measures

- **Third-party testing**: Choose herbs from suppliers who conduct independent third-party testing for purity and authenticity.
- **Know your supplier**: Establish relationships with reputable suppliers with transparent sourcing practices. Establish relationships with reputable suppliers with transparent sourcing practices.
- **Educate yourself**: Familiarize yourself with the typical appearance, smell, and taste of the herbs you use to detect potential adulteration.

Potential Allergens

Potential allergens in herbalism refer to substances within plants that can induce allergic reactions in susceptible people.

Causes

- **Proteins and secondary metabolites**: Allergens are often proteins or secondary metabolites present in plants.
- **Individual sensitivities**: Allergic reactions vary among people, and what may be safe for one person can trigger an allergic response in another.

Potential Dangers

Allergic reactions: Exposure to allergenic substances in herbs can lead to mild to severe allergic reactions ranging from skin rashes to anaphylaxis.

Preventive Measures

- **Allergy screening**: People with known allergies or sensitivities should undergo allergy screening before using new herbs.
- **Start slow**: When trying a new herb, start with a small amount to gauge the body's response.
- **Consultation with healthcare professionals**: Seek advice from healthcare professionals, especially if you have a history of allergies or are unsure about potential allergens in specific herbs.

Herbal Interactions With Medications

Herbs and herbal remedies have been used for centuries to promote health and well-being. However, it's important to know that herbs—like pharmaceutical drugs—contain active compounds that can interact with medications. These interactions may influence the effectiveness, side effects, or absorption of drugs. Understanding herb-drug interactions is vital for ensuring the safe and effective use of both herbal remedies and prescribed medications.

Factors Contributing to Herb-Drug Interactions

Pharmacokinetics

- **Absorption**: Herbs may affect the absorption of drugs in the gastrointestinal tract by altering their bioavailability.

- **Distribution**: Some herbs can impact the distribution of drugs in the bloodstream affecting their concentration in target tissues.
- **Metabolism**: Herbs may influence the enzymatic processes in the liver responsible for drug metabolism, thus, altering the rate at which drugs are broken down.
- **Excretion**: Herbs may impact the elimination of drugs from the body through affecting their duration of action.

Pharmacodynamics

- **Receptor interactions**: Active compounds in herbs may interact with receptors in the body, consequently affecting the mechanisms of action of certain drugs.
- **Enzyme inhibition or induction**: Herbs can inhibit or induce specific enzymes involved in drug metabolism, hence, altering the pharmacological effects of medications.

Individual Variability

- **Genetic factors**: Genetic variations among persons can influence how herbs and drugs are metabolized and their overall impact on the body.
- **Health status**: The presence of underlying health conditions may influence how the body responds to both herbs and drugs.

Dosage and Duration

- **Dosage levels:** The amount of herbs and drugs consumed can impact the likelihood and severity of interactions.

- **Duration of use:** Long-term use of herbs or drugs may increase the likelihood of interactions over time.

Common Herb-Drug Interactions

Anticoagulant and Antiplatelet Drugs

- **Herbs**: Garlic, ginkgo biloba, and ginger.
- **Interaction**: Increased risk of bleeding when used with anticoagulant medications like warfarin.

Blood Pressure Medications

- **Herbs**: Hawthorn, licorice, and ginseng.
- **Interaction**: Altered blood pressure control when used concurrently with antihypertensive drugs.

Immune Suppressants

- **Herbs**: Echinacea, astragalus, and goldenseal.
- **Interaction**: Potential reduction in the effectiveness of immune-suppressing medications.

Antidepressants

- **Herbs**: St. John's Wort.
- **Interaction**: Reduced efficacy of some antidepressant medications.

Diabetes Medications

- **Herbs**: Gymnema, fenugreek, and bitter melon.
- **Interaction**: Altered blood sugar control when used with antidiabetic drugs.

Preventive Measures and Best Practices

Consultation with Healthcare Professionals

- **Open communication**: Inform healthcare providers about all herbs, supplements, and medications being used.
- **Professional guidance**: Seek guidance from healthcare professionals, especially when considering herbal remedies alongside prescribed medications.

Individualized Assessment

- **Health history**: Consider the individual health status of the person, existing medical conditions, and any genetic factors that may influence interactions.
- **Monitoring**: Regular monitoring of health parameters can help identify potential interactions early.

Dosage and Duration Considerations

- **Dosage guidelines**: Follow recommended dosage guidelines for both herbs and medications.
- **Regular review**: Periodically review herbal and medication regimens with healthcare providers.

Quality and Source of Herbs

- **Reputable suppliers**: Choose herbs from reputable suppliers who adhere to quality standards.
- **Standardized extracts**: Consider using standardized herbal extracts with known concentrations of active compounds.

Patient Education

- **Informed decision-making**: Educate patients about potential interactions and empower them to make informed decisions.
- **Awareness**: Encourage people to be aware of any changes in symptoms or side effects that may signal an interaction.

Consulting With Healthcare Professionals

The Importance of Consulting Healthcare Professionals Before Using Herbal Medications

While herbs can offer numerous benefits, their use comes with potential risks and complexities. Consulting with healthcare professionals before incorporating herbal medications isn't just a recommendation but a critical step in ensuring safety, efficacy, and optimal health outcomes. Here's why consulting healthcare professionals is so vital.

Individual Health Assessment

Comprehensive Health History

Healthcare professionals assess a person's comprehensive health history, taking into account existing medical conditions, past surgeries, medications, allergies, and lifestyle factors. This thorough understanding allows them to identify potential interactions and contraindications with herbal medications.

Underlying Health Conditions

People may have underlying health conditions that can affect how the body responds to herbal remedies. Consulting healthcare professionals ensures that potential risks associated with specific health conditions are considered.

Medication Interactions

Potential Herb-Drug Interactions

Herbs can interact with prescribed medications, altering their efficacy or leading to unexpected side effects. Healthcare professionals can assess potential interactions and make necessary adjustments to medication regimens.

Dosage Adjustments

Herbal medications may require dosage adjustments when used alongside pharmaceutical drugs. Healthcare professionals can provide guidance on appropriate dosages to avoid adverse effects.

Safety and Efficacy

Safety Considerations

Healthcare professionals evaluate the safety of herbal medications, considering factors such as purity, quality, and potential contaminants. This is crucial in preventing adverse reactions and ensuring that herbal products meet quality standards.

Monitoring for Adverse Effects

Regular monitoring by healthcare professionals allows for the early detection of any adverse effects or changes in health that may be associated with herbal medication use.

Efficacy Assessment

Healthcare professionals can help people set realistic expectations regarding the efficacy of herbal medications. They provide guidance on monitoring outcomes and adjusting treatment plans as needed.

Evidence-Based Practice

Research and Evidence

Healthcare professionals rely on evidence-based practice drawing from scientific research and clinical studies to guide their recommendations. They can provide insights into the efficacy and safety of specific herbs based on the latest research findings.

Evaluation of Herbal Claims

Herbal products often come with a variety of health claims. Healthcare professionals can critically evaluate these claims by separating evidence-based benefits from anecdotal or unsupported assertions.

Tailored Recommendations

Individualized Treatment Plans

Healthcare professionals develop individualized treatment plans taking into consideration the unique needs, preferences, and health goals of each patient. This personalized approach ensures that herbal medications align with overall health strategies.

Integrative Care

Integrative healthcare involves collaboration between conventional medical approaches and complementary therapies including herbal medicine. Healthcare professionals can guide people on how to integrate herbal remedies into their overall healthcare plans.

Education and Empowerment

Informed Decision-Making

Consulting healthcare professionals empowers you to make informed decisions about their health. Professionals provide education on the potential risks and benefits of herbal medications enabling you to weigh your options wisely.

Avoiding Self-Diagnosis and Self-Treatment

Healthcare professionals discourage self-diagnosis and self-treatment with herbal remedies. Misdiagnosis or incorrect use of herbs can lead to health risks. Seeking professional guidance ensures accurate assessments and recommendations.

Legal and Ethical Considerations

Legal and Regulatory Compliance

Healthcare professionals navigate legal and regulatory frameworks related to the use of herbal medications. They provide guidance on complying with regulations ensuring the safe and legal use of herbal remedies.

Ethical Standards

Ethical considerations such as respecting individual autonomy and informed consent are integral to healthcare practice. Professionals uphold ethical standards in guiding people through decisions related to herbal medications.

Continuous Monitoring and Follow-Up

Adapting to Changes

Health conditions, medications, and individual circumstances can change over time. Healthcare professionals provide ongoing monitoring and follow-up, therefore, adapting treatment plans as needed to accommodate these changes.

Preventing Potential Risks

Regular check-ins with healthcare professionals help prevent potential risks associated with the long-term use of herbal medications. Any emerging issues can be addressed promptly.

Ethical Wild Crafting and Recognizing Cultural Origins of Herbal Practices

Ethical wild crafting, often referred to as ethical foraging or sustainable harvesting, is a practice that involves gathering wild plants and herbs in a manner that promotes ecological sustainability, respects biodiversity, and acknowledges the cultural and spiritual significance of the plants. Recognizing the cultural origins of herbal practices is an integral part of this process, as it acknowledges the traditional knowledge and wisdom passed down through generations.

Ethical Wild Crafting

Sustainable Harvesting Practices

- **Selective harvesting**: Ethical wild crafting involves selective harvesting rather than indiscriminate collection. Practitioners carefully choose specific plant parts and avoid overharvesting to allow populations to regenerate.
- **Respecting growth cycles**: Harvesting is done with consideration for the natural growth cycles of plants, thereby ensuring that they have the opportunity to complete their life cycle and reproduce.

Minimizing Environmental Impact

- **Leave-no-trace principle**: Ethical wild crafters follow the leave-no-trace principle, minimizing their impact on ecosystems and leaving the environment as undisturbed as possible.
- **Awareness of endangered species**: Practitioners stay informed about endangered or threatened plant species and avoid harvesting them.

Legal Compliance

Adherence to regulations: Ethical wild crafters are aware of and comply with local and national regulations regarding the harvesting of wild plants. This includes obtaining necessary permits and permissions.

Respect for Ecosystems

- **Maintaining biodiversity**: Ethical wild crafting practices aim to maintain biodiversity by not disrupting the balance of plant and animal species within ecosystems.
- **Caring for habitats**: Practitioners avoid damaging habitats such as wetlands or delicate ecosystems during their foraging activities.

Recognizing the Cultural Origins of Herbal Practices

Honoring Traditional Knowledge

- **Cultural heritage**: Herbal practices have deep cultural roots often spanning generations. Ethical wild crafters acknowledge and honor the traditional knowledge held by indigenous communities and local cultures.
- **Collaboration with communities**: Engaging with local communities and learning from their traditional practices fosters cultural respect and promotes sustainable relationships.

Cultural Sensitivity

- **Understanding sacred plants**: Some plants hold spiritual or sacred significance in certain cultures.

Ethical wild crafters approach these plants with cultural sensitivity, thus, respecting their sacred status.

- **Consultation with elders**: Seeking guidance and permission from indigenous elders or community leaders is a way of acknowledging and respecting cultural traditions.

Avoiding Cultural Appropriation

- **Mindful use of traditional knowledge**: Ethical wild crafters are cautious about appropriating traditional knowledge and practices. They seek permission and collaborate with communities to ensure the respectful use of traditional wisdom.
- **Attribution and acknowledgment**: When sharing information about herbal practices, ethical wild crafters acknowledge the cultural origins and sources of the knowledge they are disseminating.

Supporting Cultural Preservation

- **Community empowerment**: Ethical wild crafting practices include initiatives to support and empower local communities, subsequently contributing to the preservation of their cultural heritage.
- **Fair trade practices**: Fair trade principles are applied when purchasing herbs from communities, ensuring that the economic benefits are justly shared.

Community Education and Outreach

Public Awareness

- **Educational programs**: Ethical wild crafters engage in educational programs to raise public awareness about the importance of ethical foraging, sustainable harvesting, and the cultural origins of herbal practices.
- **Workshops and events**: Hosting workshops and events helps disseminate knowledge about both the ecological and cultural aspects of herbalism.

Advocacy for Conservation

- **Conservation initiatives**: Ethical wild crafters actively support and participate in conservation initiatives that aim to protect biodiversity, habitats, and the cultural landscapes associated with herbal practices.
- **Policy advocacy**: They may engage in advocacy efforts to promote policies that safeguard both the environment and cultural heritage.

Chapter 3

Introductory Botany for the Aspiring Herbalist

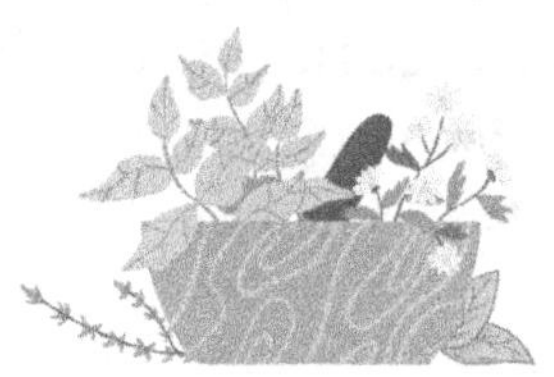

Understanding Plant Anatomy

Understanding plant anatomy is fundamental for anyone interested in herbalism, botany, gardening, or horticulture. Plants exhibit remarkable structural diversity, and each part serves specific functions critical for their growth, reproduction, and adaptation to the environment.

Roots

Structure

- **Primary root**: the main, central root that develops from the seed.
- **Secondary roots**: branching roots that emerge from the primary root.
- **Root hairs**: fine, thread-like extensions that increase the root's surface area for water and nutrient absorption.

Functions

- **Anchorage**: Roots anchor the plant in the soil, thus, providing stability.
- **Absorption**: Root hairs absorb water enriched with nutrients from the soil.
- **Storage**: Some roots store reserve food materials.

Types

- **Taproot system**: one main, dominant root with smaller lateral roots, for example, carrots and dandelion.
- **Fibrous root system**: numerous thin, shallow roots of similar diameter, for example, blueberries and sage.

Stems

Structure

- **Nodes**: points on the stem where leaves, branches, or flowers are attached.
- **Internodes**: segments between nodes.
- **Buds**: undeveloped or embryonic shoots.

Functions

- **Support**: Stems provide structural support for leaves, flowers, and fruits.
- **Transport**: Vascular bundles in stems transport water, nutrients, and sugars.
- **Photosynthesis**: Green stems can photosynthesize.

The Green Glow

Types

- **Herbaceous stems**: soft, flexible stems found in non-woody plants.
- **Woody stems**: rigid stems characterized by secondary growth and the presence of bark.

Leaves

Structure

- **Blade**: the flattened, expanded part of the leaf.
- **Petiole**: the stalk that attaches the leaf blade to the branch or stem.
- **Veins**: vascular bundles that transport water and nutrients.

Functions

- **Photosynthesis**: Chloroplasts in leaf cells capture sunlight for energy.
- **Transpiration**: Evaporation of water from leaf surfaces helps draw water from roots.
- **Gas exchange**: Stomata allow for the exchange of carbon dioxide and oxygen.

Types

- **Simple leaves**: single, undivided blades like basil and mint.
- **Compound leaves**: divided into leaflets like dill and chamomile.

Flowers

Structure

- **Receptacle**: the swollen tip of the flower stalk where floral organs attach.
- **Sepals**: outermost floral organs—usually green.
- **Petals**: brightly colored structures that attract pollinators.
- **Stamens**: male reproductive organs producing pollen.
- **Pistils**: female reproductive organs containing the ovary, style, and stigma.

Functions

- **Reproduction**: Flowers facilitate sexual reproduction by producing seeds.
- **Attracting pollinators**: Color, scent, and nectar attract pollinators like bees, butterflies, and birds.
- **Seed formation**: After pollination, fertilization occurs leading to seed development.

Types

- **Perfect flowers**: contain both male and female parts.
- **Imperfect flowers**: contain only male or female parts.
- **Complete flowers**: contain all floral organs (sepals, petals, stamens, and pistils).
- **Incomplete flowers**: lack one or more floral organs.

Introduction to Plant Classification and Families

Plant classification is a systematic approach to organizing the vast diversity of plant life on Earth. This classification based on shared characteristics and evolutionary relationships helps scientists, botanists, and enthusiasts understand the relationships between different plant species. At the broadest level, plants are classified into several major groups and each group is further divided into families.

Basic Plant Classification

Kingdom

All plants belong to the kingdom *Plantae*. They're characterized by eukaryotic cells, multicellularity, and the ability to undergo photosynthesis.

Division/Phylum

Plants are further divided into various divisions or phyla based on major morphological and reproductive characteristics. For example, the most familiar divisions are *Angiospermae* (flowering plants) and *Gymnospermae* (conifers and related plants).

Class

Within each division, plants are organized into classes based on additional shared features. In *Angiospermae*, classes include *Magnoliopsida* (dicotyledons) and *Liliopsida* (monocotyledons).

Order

Classes are further divided into orders representing groups of related families; for example, the order Rosales includes the rose family (*Rosaceae*) and others.

Family

Families consist of multiple genera with shared characteristics. For example, the family Lamiaceae includes basil, mint, sage, rosemary, bee balm, and many others. Families are the focus of our detailed exploration below.

Genus

Genera—plural of genus—group together species that share more specific characteristics.

Species

The most specific level of classification representing individual types of plants that can interbreed and produce fertile offspring.

Prominent Plant Families

Rosaceae (Rose Family)

- **Characteristics**: often include five-petaled flowers, compound leaves, and diverse fruit types.
- **Examples**: roses (*Rosa*), apples (*Malus*), strawberries (*Fragaria*).

Poaceae (Grass Family)

- **Characteristics**: typically hollow stems, parallel-veined leaves, and small, inconspicuous flowers.
- **Examples**: wheat (*Triticum*), rice (*Oryza*), bamboo (*Bambusa*).

Fabaceae (Pea Family)

- **Characteristics**: often possess compound leaves and distinctive pea-like flowers.
- **Examples**: peas (*Pisum*), beans (*Phaseolus*), clover (*Trifolium*).

Solanaceae (Nightshade Family)

- **Characteristics**: They typically have five-lobed flowers, alternate leaves, and often produce toxic alkaloids.
- **Examples**: tomatoes (*Solanum lycopersicum*), potatoes (*Solanum tuberosum*), bell peppers (*Capsicum*).

Asteraceae (Aster or Sunflower Family)

- **Characteristics**: composite flower heads (multiple tiny flowers in a central disk), often with a ring of ray flowers.
- **Examples**: sunflowers (*Helianthus*), daisies (*Bellis*), dandelions (*Taraxacum*).

Lamiaceae (Mint Family)

- **Characteristics**: square stems, opposite leaves, and aromatic oils.
- **Examples**: mint (*Mentha*), basil (*Ocimum*), rosemary (*Rosmarinus*).

Orchidaceae (Orchid Family)

- **Characteristics**: complex flowers often with a specialized lip (*labellum*) and a unique method of pollination.
- **Examples**: orchids (*Orchis*), vanilla (*Vanilla planifolia*).

Brassicaceae (Mustard or Crucifer Family)

- **Characteristics**: four-petaled flowers arranged in a cross shape often with a distinctive seed pod.

- **Examples**: cabbages (*Brassica oleracea*), mustard
  (*Brassica juncea*), radishes (*Raphanus*).

The Seasonal Lifecycle of Plants and Optimal Harvesting Times

Different stages of a plant's life offer varying concentrations of essential compounds, and harvesting at the right time ensures the best quality and yield. We'll now take a look at the four seasons and how they influence the lifecycle of plants as well as the optimal times for harvesting.

Spring

Spring is the time for perennial—enduring for many growing seasons—plants to come out of dormancy and regrow from underground roots. Annual—living for one growing season—plants sprout from seeds and seedlings emerge as temperatures rise. Plants focus on establishing roots and developing leaves in early spring.

Optimal Harvesting

- **Early spring**: Harvest young leaves and shoots for tenderness and enhanced flavor.
- **Late spring**: Flowers and buds which offer unique flavors may emerge. Harvest before they fully bloom.

Summer

Plants continue to grow focusing more on foliage and stem development. Many plants transition to the reproductive phase, producing flowers.

Optimal Harvesting

- **Early summer**: Harvest temperature-sensitive herbs and leafy greens like parsley and celery before they bolt —produce flowers—and become bitter.
- **Mid-summer**: Flowers, fruits, and vegetables are often at their peak flavor and nutritional content.
- **Late summer**: Harvest mature fruits, seeds, and late-season vegetables.

Fall

Most plants complete their growth in fall preparing for winter. Fruits and seeds ripen often ready for dispersal.

Optimal Harvesting

- **Early fall**: Continue harvesting late-season vegetables and fruits.
- **Mid-fall**: Harvest root crops and tubers before the ground freezes.
- **Late fall**: Collect seeds for propagation and storage. Some plants improve in flavor after a light frost.

Winter

Winter is a time for dormancy and rest for perennial and biennial plants. The foliage of some perennials die back completely while conserving the energy stored in their roots for the upcoming spring. The growth of evergreen plants is minimal.

In areas with milder winters, plants like sage, thyme, mint, lavender, and oregano will continue to thrive throughout the season.

Additional Considerations

Circadian Rhythms

Some plants exhibit circadian rhythms affecting the concentration of essential oils, flavors, and nutrients throughout the day. Harvesting in the morning is often recommended for optimal quality.

Lunar Phases

While not scientifically proven, some traditional farming practices consider lunar phases for planting and harvesting. The belief is that lunar cycles influence plant growth.

Weather Conditions

Weather can impact the optimal harvesting time. For example, rainy weather may dilute essential oils in herbs.

Perennial Plants

Perennial plants, which live for multiple years, may have different harvesting schedules. Harvesting times for perennial herbs like sage or thyme can be throughout the growing season.

The Basics of Wild Crafting and Sustainable Harvesting

Wild crafting is the practice of harvesting plants, herbs, and fungi from their natural environment for various purposes, such as medicinal, culinary, or craft use. However, the popularity of wild crafting brings with it the responsibility of ensuring sustainable practices to preserve ecosystems and maintain the balance of natural resources. By embracing the following ethical principles, wild crafters contribute to the preservation of natural environments, therefore, promoting a harmonious coexistence between humans and the plant kingdom.

Ethical Principles of Wild Crafting

Respect for Nature

Ethical principles ensure the sustainability and conservation of ecosystems. One fundamental principle is "leave no trace," emphasizing the importance of minimizing environmental impact. This involves avoiding damage to plants, soil, and habitats. Practitioners are encouraged to tread lightly, especially around delicate or rare species, by walking carefully to prevent trampling.

Knowledge and Education

Knowledge and education are crucial components of ethical wild crafting. Those engaged in this practice should possess a deep understanding of species identification, thoroughly learning to distinguish between plants to prevent unintentional harm to similar-looking species. Habitat awareness is also emphasized, thus, encouraging wild crafters to comprehend the ecosystems where plants grow to minimize disruption.

Legal Compliance

Legal compliance is a cornerstone of ethical wild crafting. This involves obtaining any necessary permits and adhering to local regulations governing wild crafting activities. Practitioners are urged to respect private property rights, seeking permission before harvesting on private land. This not only ensures legal compliance but also fosters positive relationships between wild crafters and landowners.

Sustainable Harvesting Practices

Through sustainable harvesting practices, people can contribute to the longevity and resilience of plant ecosystems, thus, promoting a harmonious relationship between human needs and the preservation of biodiversity.

Harvesting Techniques

Sustainable harvesting maintains the delicate balance between our consumption of plant resources and the preservation of natural ecosystems. Selective harvesting techniques play a pivotal role in this approach, hence, emphasizing the importance of choosing individual plants rather than uprooting entire populations.

Wild crafters are encouraged to employ pruning methods, selectively removing plant parts rather than removing the whole plant.

Timing and Season

Gathering plants at their optimal growth stages and considering factors such as flowering, fruiting, or root maturity ensures the preservation of plant vitality. Respecting seasons and allowing plants to complete their life cycles before harvesting further contributes to sustainable practices.

Quantity

Quantity is another crucial aspect of sustainable harvesting. Wild crafters are advised to exercise moderation, harvesting only what is necessary to avoid overexploitation of natural resources. Monitoring the health and abundance of plant populations becomes integral, with practitioners adjusting harvest quantities based on population dynamics.

Ecosystem Stewardship

Biodiversity Preservation

Preserving the biodiversity of nature is a fundamental principle in sustainable wild crafting, as it emphasizes the importance of avoiding overharvesting to maintain the ecological balance and prevent the depletion of certain plant species. It's important to protect rare or endangered plants by not harvesting them and promptly reporting sightings to conservation authorities. This contributes to the preservation of endangered or at-risk plant populations as well as the efficacy of conservation efforts.

Habitat Conservation

Habitat conservation is closely tied to biodiversity preservation. Wild crafters are advised to minimize disturbance by sticking to established trails and paths, consequently reducing habitat disruption during their foraging forays. Avoiding sensitive areas such as ecologically vulnerable habitats or protected zones is paramount to maintaining the integrity of the natural environment.

Collaboration with Indigenous Communities

Respecting traditional knowledge is a key aspect of ethical wild crafting, particularly when it involves collaboration with indigenous communities. Practitioners engaging in wild crafting practices tied to indigenous traditions should seek permission and actively collaborate with local communities. Cultural sensitivity emphasizes the importance of respecting and acknowledging the traditional knowledge of indigenous cultures concerning wild plants.

Regenerative Practices

Sustainable Cultivation

Sustainable cultivation practices promote the long-term health of both plant populations and ecosystems. One sustainable approach involves cultivating wild plants at home, hence, fostering a connection between herbalists and the plants they use. This not only provides a sustainable source but also allows herbalists to implement responsible gardening practices that do not subtract from our ecosystem.

Seed saving is another valuable technique encouraging the natural regeneration of local plant populations by allowing plants to go to seed. By supporting the reproduction cycle, wild crafters contribute to the overall health and resilience of the species they harvest.

Reforestation and Restoration

Reforestation and ecosystem restoration are integral components of sustainable wild crafting. Individuals can actively contribute to these efforts by supporting conservation initiatives focused on reforestation. By participating in or endorsing projects dedicated to restoring ecosystems, wild crafters play a role in preserving habitats and promoting the biodiversity essential for sustainable wild crafting practices.

Safety and Health Considerations

Safety and health considerations are paramount in ethical wild crafting. Purity and contamination concerns emphasize the importance of harvesting away from polluted areas, roadsides, or locations treated with pesticides. This ensures the purity of harvested plants and minimizes the risk of contaminants affecting the quality of the botanical material. Additionally, allergen awareness is crucial in identifying plants that may cause allergic reactions. Practitioners need to exercise caution when harvesting or handling such plants while prioritizing safety and health throughout their wild crafting endeavors.

Chapter 4

Essential Tools of the Trade

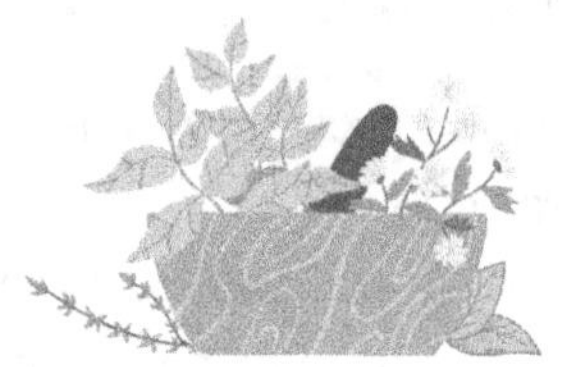

Tools Every Herbalist Needs

Herbalists rely on a variety of tools to cultivate, harvest, prepare, and administer herbs. The following tools are essential for ensuring the quality and efficacy of herbal remedies.

Gardening Tools

Pruners/Secateurs

- **Use**: harvesting leaves, flowers, and stems.
- **Benefits**: allows precise cutting without causing damage to the plant.

Harvesting Knife

- **Use**: cutting through tougher plant material such as roots or thick stems.
- **Benefits**: provides a sharp and controlled cut for efficient harvesting.

Trowel

- **Use**: digging and transplanting herbs in the garden or in containers.
- **Benefits**: helps maintain soil structure and minimizes root disturbance.

Gloves

- **Use**: protecting hands during planting, harvesting, and working with soil.
- **Benefits**: preventing skin irritation, cuts, or contact with potentially harmful plants.

Drying and Processing Tools

Drying Rack

- **Use**: air-drying herbs for preservation.
- **Benefits**: facilitates even drying and prevents mold or decay.

Dehydrator

- **Use**: speeds up the drying process for herbs.
- **Benefits**: maintains optimal temperature and humidity levels for preserving herbs.

Mortar and Pestle

- **Use**: grinding dried herbs into powder or breaking down fresh herbs.
- **Benefits**: allows for manual processing, thus, preserving the integrity of the plant.

Herb Scissors

- **Use**: cutting herbs quickly and evenly for culinary or medicinal purposes.
- **Benefits**: provides a convenient and efficient way to harvest and prepare herbs.

Measurement Tools

Digital Scale

- **Use**: weighing herbs for precise measurements in formulations.
- **Benefits**: ensures accuracy in creating herbal remedies.

Measuring Spoons

- **Use**: measuring smaller quantities of herbs or powders.
- **Benefits**: Useful for precise measurements in smaller batches.

Storage and Packaging Tools

Glass Jars

- **Use**: storing dried herbs, herbal tinctures, or infused oils.
- **Benefits**: airtight and light-resistant, subsequently preserving the quality of herbs.

Labels and Markers

- **Use**: clearly identifying herbs and formulations.
- **Benefits**: prevents confusion and ensures accurate use of herbal products.

Airtight Containers

- **Use**: storing dried herbs or herbal products.
- **Benefits**: prevents moisture and air exposure, maintaining herb quality.

Extraction Tools

Double Boiler

- **Use**: gently heating herbs in a water bath for making infusions or decoctions.
- **Benefits**: prevents direct heat, consequently preserving delicate plant compounds.

Herb Press

- **Use**: extracting liquids from herbs.
- **Benefits**: efficiently extracts herbal extracts or tinctures.

Cheesecloth or Strainer

- **Use**: straining herbal infusions or tinctures.
- **Benefits**: removes plant material resulting in a clear liquid.

Reference Materials

Herbal Books and Online Guides

- **Use**: referencing for plant identification, properties, and uses.
- **Benefits**: essential for expanding herbal knowledge and ensuring accurate information about each specific herb; many guides include how to cultivate the herbs yourself.

Traditional Tools From Diverse Cultures and Their Modern Applications

Traditional tools from diverse cultures reflect the ingenuity and resourcefulness of communities throughout history. These tools have often been crafted to address specific agricultural needs. Many of these traditional tools—rooted in cultural practices— have found modern applications either as historical artifacts or as inspiration for contemporary designs.

Japanese Hori-Hori (Soil Knife)

Traditional Use

The hori-hori was originally designed for excavating plants, cutting weeds off below the soil surface, and digging in rocky soil. It features a serrated edge for cutting roots, a concave shape for soil scooping, and a ruler for quick reference.

Modern Applications

The hori-hori is widely adopted by gardeners and landscapers for planting, weeding, and cutting. It's become a staple in modern gardening tool sets for versatility.

Chinese Iron Plow

Traditional Use

The iron plow was introduced during the Han dynasty for agricultural purposes and consisted of an iron plowshare with a horizontal wooden shaft.

Modern Applications

The Chinese iron plow evolved into modern plow designs used in agriculture worldwide. It contributed to the development of mechanized plows for efficient large-scale farming.

Mattock

Traditional Use

The exact origin of the mattock is unknown, but it's been used for digging, chopping, and breaking up soil since before the bronze age.

Modern Application

It remains useful for heavy-duty tasks in hard soil, thickly matted sod, as well as larger gardens.

Olla

Traditional Use

An olla is a watering tool of Native American origin. It's a clay pot that is buried in the soil for slow and consistent watering.

Modern Application

Many modern permutations of the olla remain on the market to this day. It's an eco-friendly and water-saving irrigation method, particularly useful in arid regions.

Birch Bark Containers

Traditional Use

Native Americans used birch bark containers for storing a vast array of items including herbs to preserve their aroma, flavor, and potency.

Modern Application

In modern times, they're mostly used for decoration and are an eco-friendly alternative to plastic.

Sickle

Traditional Use

Sickle blades came into use in Southwest Asia when our ancestors transitioned from hunter-gatherers to an agrarian culture.

Modern Application

Sickles are still used for efficient cutting of herbs and plants because of their simplicity and low-cost.

Properly Storing Herbs to Retain Potency

Proper storage is essential to keep herbs fresh and retain their potency. Both freshly harvested and purchased herbs can lose flavor, aroma, and medicinal properties if not stored correctly. We'll now take a look at the different ways to properly store herbs for optimal freshness:

Harvest or Purchase Fresh Quality Herbs

Harvest at the Right Time

- Harvest herbs when essential oils are at their peak usually in the morning after the dew has dried.
- Choose leaves and flowers that are free from pests or diseases.

Select High-Quality Purchased Herbs

- When buying herbs, choose fresh-looking, vibrant leaves without discoloration or wilting.
- Prefer organic or locally sourced herbs for better quality.

Cleaning and Drying

Gentle Cleaning

- Rinse herbs gently under cold water to remove dirt or insects.
- Pat them dry with a clean cloth or use a salad spinner to remove excess water.

Air-Drying

- Air-dry herbs like rosemary, thyme, or oregano by bundling them and hanging them upside down in a dry, well-ventilated area.
- Avoid direct sunlight to prevent the breakdown of essential oils.

Dehydrating

- Use a dehydrator for herbs like basil, parsley, or mint. Follow the dehydrator's instructions for temperature and time.
- Alternatively, use an oven set to low heat for dehydrating.

Proper Storage Containers

Airtight Glass Jars

- Store dried herbs in clean, dry, airtight glass jars.
- Avoid plastic containers, as they may not provide an airtight seal.

Dark Containers

- Choose dark-colored glass jars to protect herbs from light exposure.
- Light can degrade essential oils and affect the flavor and potency of herbs.

Storage Location

Cool and Dark Environment

- Store herbs in a cool, dark place, away from direct sunlight and heat.
- Avoid storing herbs near the stove or other heat sources.

Refrigeration or Freezing

- While some herbs do well in the refrigerator (e.g., cilantro, parsley), others can be frozen in ice cube trays with water or oil (e.g., basil, chives).
- Freezing is ideal for preserving the fresh taste of delicate herbs.

Labeling and Organization

Label Jars Clearly

- Label each jar with the name of the herb and the date of harvesting or purchase.
- This helps you keep track of important information like what herb it contains, its potency, the date and time of harvest, and parts of the plant used.

Keep Similar Herbs Together

- Group herbs with similar storage requirements together.
- For example, store delicate herbs like cilantro and parsley together; sturdier herbs like rosemary and thyme can be stored together.

Avoid Crushing Until Use

Whole or Coarsely Ground

- Keep herbs in their whole or coarsely ground form until you're ready to use them.
- Grinding or crushing just before use helps retain the maximum flavor and potency.

Regular Check and Rotation

Check for Freshness

- Regularly inspect stored herbs for any signs of mold, discoloration, or loss of aroma.
- Remove any spoiled or deteriorated herbs to prevent contamination.

Rotate Stock

- Use the "first in, first out" principle to ensure you're using the oldest herbs first.
- Rotate your herb stock regularly to maintain freshness.

Herb Preservation Techniques

Infused Oils or Vinegars

- Create infused oils or vinegars with fresh herbs for extended shelf life and diverse culinary uses.
- Keep these creations in dark bottles and refrigerate for longevity.

Herb Butter

- Make herb-infused butter by blending chopped herbs with softened butter.
- Form the mixture into a log, wrap in parchment paper, and freeze for later use.

Chapter 5

Getting to Know Key Herbs

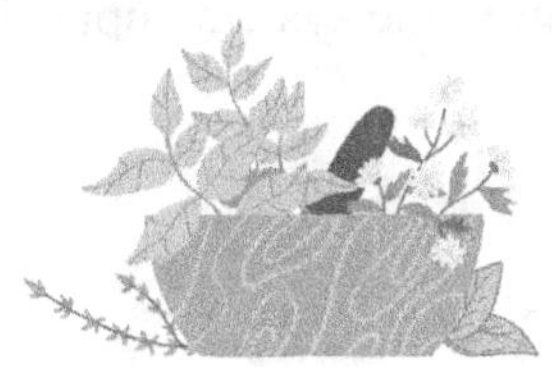

Aloe Vera (*Aloe barbadensis*)

Aloe vera is a staple in global skincare and wellness practices. Its versatile uses and cultural symbolism make it a revered botanical worldwide.

Uses

Topical Applications

- **Skin soothing**: Aloe vera gel—derived from the succulent plant's leaves—is a renowned topical remedy. Its cooling effect and moisturizing properties make it effective for sunburn relief, faster wound healing, and managing skin conditions like eczema and psoriasis.
- **Anti-inflammatory**: The gel's anti-inflammatory components provide relief for insect bites, rashes, and minor burns.

Oral Consumption

- **Digestive support**: Aloe vera juice—made from aloe gel—is consumed for its digestive benefits. It aids in alleviating constipation and promoting a healthy gut.
- **Overall wellness**: Some enthusiasts use aloe vera supplements for immune system support and overall well-being.

Properties

- **Anti-inflammatory**: Aloe vera contains compounds like bradykinase that offer natural anti-inflammatory effects.
- **Antioxidant**: Rich in antioxidants including vitamins A, C, and E, aloe vera helps combat oxidative stress and promote skin health.
- **Antimicrobial**: Aloe vera contains salicylates, which are naturally antimicrobial and contribute to its effectiveness in wound healing and skin care.

Other properties include anticancer, antidiabetic, and antihyperlipidemic (fat lowering) effects.

History and Cultural Significance

Aloe vera's historical use traces back to ancient civilizations. Egyptians referred to it as the "plant of immortality," and Cleopatra is said to have used it for skin care. Greeks and Romans documented its healing properties and employed it for wounds and various ailments.

Aloe vera found its place in traditional medicine across cultures from Ayurveda in India to TCM. It was valued for its diverse therapeutic applications.

In the 20th century, scientific exploration delved into aloe vera's chemical composition. This led to its commercialization in skincare products, pharmaceuticals, and dietary supplements.

Anise (*Pimpinella anisum*)

Anise with its aromatic allure and therapeutic virtues has left an indelible mark on the landscape of herbal remedies.

Uses

Topical Applications

- **Respiratory aid**: Anise's aromatic properties make it useful in topical applications for respiratory issues. Anise oil is sometimes diluted and applied to the chest for relief from congestion.
- **Skin care**: Anise's antimicrobial and anti-inflammatory attributes contribute to its use in skin care, thus, addressing issues like acne and inflammation.

Oral Consumption

- **Digestive health**: Anise is commonly used orally to alleviate digestive discomfort acting as a carminative to reduce bloating and aid in digestion.
- **Culinary uses**: Anise seeds are employed in cooking, as they add a distinctive flavor to dishes and desserts.

Properties

- **Antimicrobial**: Anise possesses natural antimicrobial properties making it beneficial for addressing skin issues and potential internal microbial imbalances.

- **Carminative**: Anise's carminative properties contribute to its effectiveness in easing digestive discomfort and reducing bloating and flatulence.
- **Aromatic compounds**: Anise is rich in aromatic compounds such as anethole which is anti-inflammatory, anticarcinogenic, antidiabetic, immunomodulatory, neuroprotective, and antithrombotic.

History and Cultural Significance

Anise has ancient roots with evidence of its use in ancient Egypt, Greece, and Rome. It was esteemed for its aromatic qualities and potential medicinal benefits. The ancient Greek physician Dioscorides documented anise's use in herbal medicine.

Anise has been incorporated into various traditional medicine systems for its digestive and respiratory benefits including Ayurveda and TCM.

Anise continued to be a prominent herb in medieval and Renaissance herbalism. Monastic gardens in medieval Europe often cultivated anise for its medicinal properties.

Moreover, during the Renaissance herbalists like Nicholas Culpeper acknowledged anise's digestive benefits.

Ashwagandha (*Withania somnifera*)

Ashwagandha is deeply rooted in Ayurvedic traditions and has transcended its historical origins to become globally recognized.

Uses

Topical Applications

Skin health: Ashwagandha, is believed to promote skin health when used topically. Its anti-inflammatory and antioxidant properties may aid in managing skin conditions and maintaining a healthy complexion.

Oral Consumption

- **Adaptogenic benefits**: Ashwagandha is primarily consumed orally as an adaptogenic herb. It is known to help the body adapt to stress, hence, supporting the nervous system and promoting overall well-being.
- **Energy and vitality**: Traditional use involves ashwagandha as a tonic to enhance energy levels, vitality, and physical stamina.

Properties

- **Adaptogenic**: Ashwagandha is classified as an adaptogen helping the body manage stress by regulating the physiological response to various stressors.
- **Anti-inflammatory**: Its anti-inflammatory properties contribute to its potential role in managing inflammatory conditions and promoting joint health.
- **Immunomodulatory**: Ashwagandha's immunomodulatory effects may support a balanced immune system, therefore, helping the body respond appropriately to immune challenges.
- **Cognitive support**: Studies indicate that ashwagandha may support cognitive function and memory, thus, making it potentially of interest for brain health.

History and Cultural Significance

Ashwagandha has a robust history in Ayurvedic medicine. It is considered a Rasayana—an herb that promotes longevity and rejuvenation. It is often referred to as Indian ginseng.

Ashwagandha holds cultural significance in India. It is considered a key herb for promoting vitality and resilience.

Asian Ginseng (*Panax ginseng*)

Ginseng has gained global popularity as a natural remedy featured in various dietary supplements and wellness products.

Uses

Topical Applications

Skin care: While not commonly used topically, some formulations include ginseng for potential skin benefits. It is believed to possess anti-aging properties that promote skin elasticity and vitality.

Oral Consumption

- **Adaptogenic tonic**: Asian Ginseng is primarily consumed orally for its adaptogenic properties. It is hailed as a tonic that helps the body adapt to stress, thus, enhancing overall resilience.
- **Energy and vitality**: Often taken as a supplement, ginseng is believed to boost energy levels, improve stamina, and combat fatigue.
- **Cognitive health**: Ginseng is explored for its potential cognitive benefits including improved memory and concentration.

Properties

- **Adaptogenic**: Asian Ginseng is renowned for its adaptogenic nature, assisting the body in coping with stress and maintaining balance.
- **Immunomodulatory**: Research suggests that ginseng may have immunomodulatory effects supporting a healthy immune system.
- **Antioxidant**: Ginsenosides, the active compounds in ginseng, exhibit antioxidant properties aiding in the neutralization of free radicals.

History and Cultural Significance

Asian Ginseng has an extensive history in TCM dating back thousands of years. It is classified as a superior herb revered for promoting longevity and vitality. It was mentioned in the ancient Chinese medical text the *Shennong Ben Cao Jing*.

Astragalus (*Astragalus membranaceus*)

Also known as Milkvetch, astragalus has found a place in modern herbalism embraced for its holistic benefits and contributions to well-being.

Uses

Oral Consumption

- **Immune support**: Astragalus is revered for its immune-modulating properties, supporting the body's defense mechanisms against infections.
- **Adaptogenic tonic**: Consumed as a tonic, astragalus is recognized for its adaptogenic nature, as it helps the body adapt to stress and promoting resilience.

- **Energy and vitality**: It is often incorporated into formulations to enhance energy levels, combat fatigue, and promote overall vitality.

Properties

- **Immunomodulatory**: Astragalus is renowned for its immunomodulatory effects stimulating and regulating the immune system for optimal function.
- **Adaptogenic**: Classified as an adaptogen, astragalus helps the body adapt to stressors by promoting a balanced response to physical and mental challenges.
- **Anti-inflammatory**: Studies suggest anti-inflammatory properties contributing to its potential in managing inflammatory conditions.

History and Cultural Significance

Astragalus holds a prominent place in TCM where it is known as huáng qí. It is classified as a Qi-tonifying herb nourishing the vital energy of the body.

Astragalus was traditionally used to invigorate the spleen and lungs, as documented in ancient texts like the Shennong Bencaojing.

Bilberry (*Vaccinium myrtillus*)

Bilberry supplements are popular in the wellness industry offering a concentrated form of the herb for those seeking antioxidant support and potential vision benefits. It is also known as European Blueberry.

Uses

Topical Applications

- **Eye health**: Bilberry is often used topically in formulations aimed at promoting eye health. Its antioxidant properties may support the delicate structures of the eyes and alleviate eye fatigue.
- **Skin care**: Some skincare products incorporate bilberry for its antioxidant content, hence, contributing to skin health.

Oral Consumption

- **Vision support**: Traditionally, bilberry is consumed orally for its benefits to vision. It is believed to enhance night vision and support overall eye health.
- **Antioxidant boost**: Bilberry is valued for its high anthocyanin content, thereby acting as a potent antioxidant that may combat oxidative stress in the body.

Properties

- **Antioxidant-rich**: Bilberry's deep purple color is attributed to anthocyanins—potent antioxidants that neutralize free radicals and contribute to its potential health benefits.
- **Anthocyanosides**: These specific compounds in bilberry are associated with vascular health and may support capillary strength and integrity.
- **Anti-inflammatory**: Studies suggest anti-inflammatory properties potentially contributing to the herb's role in managing inflammatory conditions.

History and Cultural Significance

Bilberry gained recognition during World War II when British Royal Air Force pilots reportedly consumed bilberry jam to enhance their night vision. While the accuracy of this legend is debated, it contributed to bilberry's reputation for supporting vision.

Bilberry has a rich history in European herbal traditions. It was used in traditional folk medicine for various conditions including digestive issues and urinary tract complaints.

Bitter Orange (*Citrus aurantium*)

Other names include Seville orange and Marmalade orange.

Uses

Topical Applications

- **Aromatherapy**: Bitter orange essential oil—derived from the peel—is used in aromatherapy for its invigorating and uplifting scent. It is believed to have mood-enhancing properties.
- **Skin care**: Some skincare products incorporate bitter orange for its astringent properties, therefore, potentially aiding in balancing oily skin.

Oral Consumption

- **Digestive aid**: Bitter orange has been traditionally used to stimulate digestion with the fruit and peel sometimes consumed in herbal formulations or teas.
- **Weight management**: Bitter orange extract is found in some weight loss supplements due to its purported role in promoting metabolism and fat burning.

Properties

- **Citrus aroma**: Bitter orange's aromatic properties contribute to its use in aromatherapy providing a refreshing and invigorating scent.
- **Astringent**: The astringent qualities of bitter orange are used in skin care where it may help tone and tighten the skin.
- **Alkaloids and synephrine**: Bitter orange contains alkaloids including synephrine, which is associated with potential stimulant effects and its role in weight management formulations.

History and Cultural Significance

Bitter orange has a history of use in TCM and Ayurvedic medicine. It was employed for various purposes including digestive support and respiratory health.

In Ayurveda, bitter orange was sometimes used to address conditions related to excess Kapha dosha.

In some cultures, bitter orange trees are considered symbols of prosperity and good fortune. The fragrant blossoms are used in traditional celebrations and ceremonies. The fruit has been used in culinary traditions for its distinct flavor. The peel is often candied, and the fruit is used in marmalades and beverages.

Black Cohosh (*Actaea racemosa*)

Black cohosh stands as an herbal ally rooted in Native American traditions and embraced for its role in women's health.

Uses

Topical Applications

Muscle relaxation: Some topical formulations containing black cohosh are used for their potential muscle-relaxing properties. These may be applied to areas experiencing tension or discomfort.

Oral Consumption

- **Menopausal symptom relief**: Black cohosh is predominantly consumed orally to address menopausal symptoms such as hot flashes, night sweats, and mood fluctuations. It is a popular herbal remedy among women seeking natural alternatives to hormonal therapies.
- **Menstrual support**: Traditionally, black cohosh has been used for menstrual irregularities and to ease discomfort associated with the menstrual cycle.

Properties

- **Phytoestrogenic activity**: Black cohosh is believed to have phytoestrogenic properties acting as a plant-based estrogen substitute. This is thought to contribute to its efficacy in managing menopausal symptoms.
- **Anti-inflammatory**: Studies suggest that black cohosh may possess anti-inflammatory properties potentially contributing to its use for conditions involving inflammation.
- **Serotonergic effects**: The herb is thought to interact with serotonin receptors, which may influence mood regulation and contribute to its use for emotional well-being.

History and Cultural Significance

Black cohosh has a long history of use among Native American communities, particularly by the Algonquian-speaking tribes. It was valued for its various medicinal properties, including its potential as a women's health remedy.

The Cherokee and Iroquois tribes used black cohosh for gynecological concerns and to address rheumatism. Some Native American tribes incorporated black cohosh into rituals and ceremonies. It was believed to have spiritual significance, particularly in rites related to women's well-being.

European settlers learned about black cohosh from Native Americans and adopted its use for women's health in the 19th century. It became a staple in early American herbalism.

During the women's health movement in the 20th century, black cohosh gained popularity as a natural remedy for menopausal symptoms. It was embraced as an alternative to synthetic hormones.

Butterbur (*Petasites hybridus*)

Butterbur's integration into modern health practices symbolizes the evolving landscape of herbalism. As a scientifically validated remedy for migraines, it reflects the merging of traditional wisdom with contemporary healthcare approaches.

Uses

Topical Applications

Skin conditions: Some topical formulations containing butterbur extract are explored for their potential in addressing skin conditions. The anti-inflammatory properties may contribute to its topical use.

Oral Consumption

- **Migraine prevention**: Butterbur is primarily consumed orally for migraine prevention. It is recognized for its potential to reduce the frequency and severity of migraines.
- **Allergy relief**: Traditionally, butterbur has been used for allergy relief, especially in managing symptoms like sneezing and nasal congestion.
- **Anti-inflammatory**: Its anti-inflammatory properties extend to internal use, hence, making it valuable for conditions involving inflammation.

Properties

- **Petasins**: Butterbur contains petasins—compounds believed to contribute to its anti-inflammatory effects. These may play a role in alleviating migraines and other inflammatory conditions.
- **Antispasmodic**: Butterbur is recognized for its antispasmodic properties, which may help relax smooth muscle tissue and contribute to its use in managing migraines.
- **Allergen inhibition**: Some studies suggest that butterbur may inhibit the production of certain chemicals involved in the allergic response, thus, supporting its use for allergy relief.

History and Cultural Significance

Butterbur has a history of use in traditional European herbalism, where it was employed for various medicinal purposes including the treatment of headaches and respiratory conditions. In Germany, it became an approved treatment for migraines.

Butterbur gained prominence in the late 20th century for its efficacy in migraine management. Clinical studies supported its role in reducing the frequency and intensity of migraines.

Cat's Claw (*Uncaria tomentosa*)

Cat's claw is commonly found in herbal supplements and tinctures, offering a convenient way for people to harness its potential health benefits.

Uses

Topical Applications

- **Wound healing**: Cat's claw has been used topically for wound healing in traditional practices. Its anti-inflammatory properties may contribute to skin recovery.
- **Arthritis relief**: Some topical formulations are explored for arthritis relief due to the herb's potential anti-inflammatory effects.

Oral Consumption

- **Immune support**: Cat's claw is often consumed orally for immune system support. It is believed to enhance immune function and defend against infections.
- **Anti-inflammatory**: The herb is recognized for its anti-inflammatory properties, making it a popular choice for managing inflammatory conditions.
- **Digestive health**: Cat's claw is used to support digestive health addressing conditions such as gastritis and other gastrointestinal issues.

Properties

- **Alkaloids**: Cat's claw contains alkaloids including oxindole and tetracyclic alkaloids, which are associated with its immunomodulatory effects.
- **Antioxidant**: The presence of antioxidants in Cat's claw contributes to its ability to neutralize free radicals, potentially aiding in overall health.
- **Anti-inflammatory**: Cat's claw's anti-inflammatory properties are attributed to its ability to inhibit certain inflammatory pathways, thus, offering relief for conditions like arthritis.

History and Cultural Significance

Indigenous communities in the Amazon rainforest have a rich history of using Cat's claw for various health purposes. It is traditionally regarded as a powerful medicinal plant. Tribes like the Asháninka and the Aguaruna have used Cat's claw for generations to address a spectrum of ailments.

Cat's claw holds significance in shamanic and spiritual practices among Amazonian tribes. It is often used in rituals and ceremonies, as it is believed to have protective and purifying qualities.

Chamomile—German and Roman (*Matricaria chamomilla* and *Chamaemelum nobile*)

Chamomile is a key ingredient in a variety of commercial products including teas, essential oils, skincare items, and herbal supplements.

Uses

Topical Applications

- **Skin irritations**: Chamomile's anti-inflammatory and soothing properties make it beneficial for topical use on skin irritations, rashes, and minor wounds.
- **Eye compresses**: Chamomile tea bags are often used in compresses to soothe tired eyes and reduce puffiness.

Oral Consumption

- **Digestive aid**: Chamomile tea is consumed orally for its digestive benefits, as it alleviates indigestion, bloating, and gas.
- **Relaxation and sleep**: Chamomile is renowned for its calming effects, therefore, it is a popular choice for promoting relaxation and improving sleep.

Properties

- **Anti-inflammatory**: Chamomile's anti-inflammatory properties are attributed to compounds like chamazulene, which helps reduce inflammation both internally and externally.
- **Calming and relaxing**: Chamomile contains apigenin—a compound known for its calming effects on the nervous system—contributing to its role in relaxation and sleep support.
- **Antioxidant**: The presence of antioxidants in chamomile helps combat oxidative stress contributing to its overall health benefits.

History and Cultural Significance

Chamomile has a long history dating back to ancient Egypt and Rome where it was used for its medicinal properties. It was revered for its soothing and healing effects.

In traditional European herbalism, chamomile gained popularity for its ability to calm digestive discomfort and promote restful sleep. It was commonly used in infusions, salves, and baths.

Chamomile symbolizes tranquility and relaxation across cultures. Its association with calmness has contributed to its cultural significance in rituals and ceremonies centered on well-being.

Chasteberry (*Vitex agnus-castus*)

Chasteberry found its place in traditional herbalism, particularly in supporting women's health.

Uses

Topical Applications

Skin conditions: Chasteberry, may be used for managing certain skin conditions when applied topically. Its anti-inflammatory properties can contribute to skin health.

Oral Consumption

- **Hormonal balance**: Chasteberry is predominantly consumed orally to support hormonal balance in women. It is often used to alleviate symptoms of premenstrual syndrome (PMS), irregular menstruation, and menopausal discomfort.
- **Fertility support**: Traditionally, chasteberry has been associated with promoting female reproductive health

including supporting fertility and addressing conditions like polycystic ovary syndrome (PCOS).

Properties

- **Hormone regulation**: Chasteberry is believed to influence the hormonal balance by acting on the pituitary gland. It may modulate the secretion of hormones like prolactin and luteinizing hormone.
- **Dopaminergic effects**: The herb has dopaminergic effects i.e., it influences dopamine levels. This action is thought to contribute to its role in alleviating symptoms related to hormonal fluctuations.
- **Anti-inflammatory**: Chasteberry's anti-inflammatory properties potentially aid in conditions where inflammation is a contributing factor.

History and Cultural Significance

Chasteberry has historical roots in ancient Greece and Rome where it was used to suppress libido (hence the name "chasteberry"). It was associated with the goddess Hera, thus, emphasizing fidelity.

In medieval Europe, chasteberry gained recognition for its purported ability to support chastity. Monks would chew the berries to suppress sexual desire, so it became known as the "monk's pepper."

Cinnamon (*Cinnamomum verum* and *Cinnamomum cassia*)

Cinnamon supplements are popular for those seeking its health benefits, especially for blood sugar management.

Uses

Topical Applications

- **Skin care**: Cinnamon—with its antimicrobial properties—can be used topically to address certain skin issues such as acne. However, caution is advised due to its potential skin sensitivity.
- **Hair health**: Cinnamon may be applied to the scalp or incorporated into hair masks for benefits including improved circulation and scalp health.

Oral Consumption

- **Digestive aid**: Cinnamon is renowned for its digestive benefits. Consuming it in teas or adding it to dishes may help alleviate indigestion and support overall digestive health.
- **Blood sugar management**: Cinnamon is studied for its potential role in managing blood sugar levels, thus, making it beneficial for people with diabetes or those looking to regulate glucose.

Properties

- **Antioxidant-rich**: Cinnamon is rich in antioxidants—particularly polyphenols—which help combat oxidative stress and inflammation.
- **Anti-inflammatory**: The spice possesses anti-inflammatory properties contributing to its potential in managing inflammatory conditions.
- **Antimicrobial**: Cinnamon's antimicrobial properties make it valuable for addressing bacterial and fungal issues.

History and Cultural Significance

Cinnamon has a storied history dating back to ancient times. It was highly prized along trade routes with its origins shrouded in mystery. It was brought from the East to the West through intricate trade networks.

Cinnamon was used in ancient Egypt for embalming and as a spice. It was also highly sought after in Rome where it was considered a luxury item.

Cinnamon has been a staple in traditional medicine across cultures. It was used for various ailments including respiratory issues, digestive complaints, and as a warming remedy.

Cranberry (*Vaccinium macrocarpon*)

Cranberry sauce is a staple in Thanksgiving meals in the United States symbolizing gratitude and abundance. Its vibrant color and tart flavor complement a variety of dishes from sauces and jams to baked goods.

Uses

Topical Applications

- **Skin care**: Cranberry—rich in antioxidants—can be applied topically to the skin. Its potential antibacterial properties may contribute to skincare routines and in addressing conditions like acne.
- **Hair health**: Cranberry extracts or juices are sometimes used in hair treatments for potential benefits like improved scalp health.

Oral Consumption

- **Urinary tract health**: Cranberry is renowned for its role in promoting urinary tract health. Consuming cranberry products is believed to help prevent urinary tract infections (UTIs).
- **Antioxidant boost**: The high antioxidant content of cranberries makes them a valuable addition to the diet, contributing to overall health.

Properties

- **Proanthocyanidins**: Cranberries contain proanthocyanidins—compounds that may prevent bacteria, particularly E. coli, from adhering to the urinary tract walls.
- **Antioxidant-rich**: The fruit is rich in antioxidants including vitamin C, quercetin, and resveratrol, which contribute to its ability to combat oxidative stress.
- **Anti-inflammatory**: Cranberry's anti-inflammatory properties may extend benefits beyond urinary health, therefore, potentially contributing to overall inflammation reduction.

History and Cultural Significance

Native American tribes were among the first to use cranberries for their medicinal and nutritional value. They used them as food, dyes, and in poultices for wound healing. The Wampanoag people introduced cranberries to early European settlers, thus, fostering the fruit's integration into colonial diets.

Folk medicine traditions embraced cranberries for various ailments from digestive issues to wound healing. It earned a place in early pharmacopeias for its diverse applications.

Sailors later consumed cranberries to prevent scurvy due to their vitamin C content. This historical use emphasized the fruit's nutritional significance.

Dandelion (*Taraxacum officinale*)

Dandelion, often dismissed as a weed, emerges as a powerhouse in herbalism and culinary arts. As a symbol of resilience and a provider of nourishment, dandelion adds its golden touch to the vibrant tapestry of herbal traditions.

Uses

Topical Applications

- **Skin care**: Dandelion sap—derived from the stem—has been traditionally used topically to address skin issues like warts and eczema.
- **Salves and balms**: Dandelion-infused salves and balms may be applied to soothe dry or irritated skindue to its anti-inflammatory properties.

Oral Consumption

- **Digestive aid**: Dandelion is consumed orally as a digestive aid. Its bitter compounds stimulate digestion, thus, supporting liver and gallbladder function.
- **Diuretic effects**: Dandelion is a natural diuretic promoting urine production and potentially aiding in detoxification.
- **Nutritional boost**: Dandelion greens are rich in vitamins and minerals, thus, contributing to overall nutrition when included in salads or cooked dishes.

Properties

- **Bitter compounds**: The bitter compounds in dandelion like taraxacin stimulate digestive processes, as they enhance the production of digestive juices.
- **Diuretic action**: Dandelion's diuretic effects are attributed to compounds that increase urine production, therefore, potentially aiding in detoxification.
- **Antioxidant-rich**: Dandelion is rich in antioxidants offering protection against oxidative stress including beta-carotene and polyphenols.

History and Cultural Significance

Dandelion has a rich history in traditional medicine. Various cultures used it to address ailments like digestive issues, liver problems, and skin conditions. Native American and European herbal traditions embraced dandelion for its diverse medicinal properties. Considered a versatile herb in TCM, it is used for its potential to reduce inflammation and remove toxins from the body.

Dandelion greens have been part of culinary traditions and are used in salads, soups, and teas. They were historically foraged and included in diets for their nutritional value.

Echinacea (*Echinacea angustifolia, Echinacea pallida,* and *Echinacea purpurea*)

Echinacea supplements including capsules, tinctures, and teas are widely available. They are commonly used during cold and flu seasons for immune support.

Uses

Topical Applications

- **Skin health**: Echinacea is sometimes used topically for skin health. Creams or salves with echinacea extract may be applied to promote wound healing and reduce inflammation.
- **Skin conditions**: Some people use echinacea topically to address skin conditions like eczema and psoriasis.

Oral Consumption

- **Immune support**: Echinacea is primarily consumed orally to support the immune system. It is believed to stimulate the body's defense mechanisms hence, aiding in the prevention and recovery from infections.
- **Respiratory health**: Echinacea is often taken to alleviate symptoms of respiratory infections such as the common cold or flu.

Properties

- **Immunostimulant**: Echinacea is renowned for its immunostimulant properties enhancing the activity of immune cells like macrophages and stimulating the production of cytokines.
- **Anti-inflammatory**: The herb exhibits anti-inflammatory effects contributing to its potential in reducing inflammation and easing symptoms of infections.
- **Antioxidant-rich**: Echinacea is rich in antioxidants including flavonoids, which help combat oxidative stress and support overall health.

History and Cultural Significance

Native American tribes, particularly the Plains Indians, used echinacea for various purposes including wound healing and addressing respiratory issues. Its use was introduced to early European settlers by Native American healers.

Elderberry (*Sambucus nigra*)

Elderberry has found its place in modern wellness practices with people incorporating it into their daily routines for immune-boosting benefits.

Uses

Topical Applications

- **Skin health**: Elderberry—with its antioxidant properties —may be applied topically to support skin health. It is believed to offer protection against oxidative stress and promote a healthy complexion.
- **Wound healing**: Some traditional practices involve using elderberry salves or ointments for wound healing, thus, leveraging its anti-inflammatory effects.

Oral Consumption

- **Immune support**: Elderberry is primarily consumed orally for immune support. It is believed to stimulate the immune system, especially during cold and flu seasons.
- **Respiratory health**: Elderberry syrup or extracts are often taken to alleviate symptoms of respiratory infections such as coughs and congestion.

Properties

- **Antiviral activity**: Elderberry is known for its antiviral properties, particularly against certain strains of influenza viruses. It may inhibit the replication of viruses.
- **Rich in antioxidants**: The berries are rich in antioxidants including flavonoids, which help neutralize free radicals and contribute to overall health.
- **Anti-inflammatory**: Elderberry exhibits anti-inflammatory effects, thereby potentially reducing inflammation and easing symptoms of respiratory infections.

History and Cultural Significance

Elderberry has a rich history in folk medicine traditions, especially in Europe. It was used for a variety of ailments from colds and fevers to rheumatic conditions. Elderberry was esteemed for its medicinal properties and was often referred to as the "medicine chest" of the country people. Traditionally, elderberry wine or cordials were crafted for their health benefits.

Native American tribes also used elderberry for medicinal purposes. The plant was respected for its versatility in addressing different health concerns.

European Mistletoe (*Viscum album*)

Mistletoe extracts are sometimes used as complementary therapies for cancer patients, especially in certain European countries where mistletoe therapy is more widely accepted.

The Green Glow

Uses

Topical Applications

- **Arthritis and joint pain**: Some traditional practices involve using mistletoe topically to alleviate arthritis and joint pain. Ointments or compresses may be applied to affected areas.
- **Wound healing**: Mistletoe extracts may be applied topically to wounds believed to promote healing and prevent infections.

Oral Consumption

- **Cancer therapy**: Mistletoe has been used orally as an alternative cancer therapy. Some proponents believe it may stimulate the immune system and exhibit cytotoxic effects on cancer cells.
- **Cardiovascular health**: In traditional herbalism, mistletoe has been used for cardiovascular health with suggestions of benefits for blood pressure regulation.

Properties

- **Immune modulation**: Mistletoe is believed to modulate the immune system by enhancing its activity against infections and potentially supporting the body's defenses.
- **Cytotoxic effects**: Compounds in mistletoe have been studied for their potential cytotoxic effects on cancer cells, thus, making mistletoe a subject of interest in integrative cancer care.
- **Cardiovascular effects**: Some studies suggest mistletoe may have cardiovascular benefits including vasodilatory

effects that could contribute to blood pressure regulation.

History and Cultural Significance

Mistletoe has symbolic importance in Druidic traditions where it was considered a sacred plant with healing properties. Druids believed mistletoe could ward off evil and promote well-being. In some rituals, mistletoe was cut with a golden sickle and used for various purposes, including healing.

In Celtic and Norse mythology, mistletoe was associated with fertility, protection, and healing. These cultures viewed it as a symbol of life and rebirth. The tradition of kissing under the mistletoe during the winter holiday season has its roots in these ancient customs.

European herbalists historically used mistletoe for various ailments including epilepsy, infertility, and cardiovascular issues. It was valued for its mystical and medicinal qualities.

Evening Primrose (*Oenothera biennis*)

Evening primrose gained popularity in the 20th century as a natural remedy. Its use expanded with the recognition of gamma-linolenic acid's (GLA's) benefits and its potential in addressing women's health issues. It is a common ingredient in skincare formulations including creams, serums, and oils.

Uses

Topical Applications

- **Skin health**: Evening primrose oil (EPO) is often applied topically for skin health. Its GLA content is believed to benefit conditions like eczema and dermatitis.

- **Anti-aging**: EPO is used in skin care for its potential anti-aging effects. Its moisturizing properties may contribute to skin elasticity and a youthful complexion.

Oral Consumption

- **Women's health**: Evening primrose is commonly used orally for women's health, particularly to alleviate symptoms of PMS and menopause.
- **Inflammatory conditions**: EPO is taken for its anti-inflammatory properties, as it's potentially beneficial for conditions like arthritis and joint pain.

Properties

- **GLA**: Evening primrose oil is rich in GLA—an essential fatty acid. GLA is known for its anti-inflammatory effects and its role in supporting skin and joint health.
- **Hormonal balance**: Evening primrose is believed to help regulate hormonal balance, thereby making it a popular choice for women experiencing hormonal fluctuations during different life stages.
- **Antioxidant content**: The oil contains antioxidants contributing to its potential in combating oxidative stress and promoting overall well-being.

History and Cultural Significance

Native American tribes historically used evening primrose for various ailments. The plant was valued for its medicinal properties and different tribes had specific uses for different parts of the plant.

In European herbal traditions, evening primrose gained recognition for its therapeutic potential. It was often used for skin conditions, respiratory issues, and women's health.

Fenugreek (*Trigonella foenum-graecum*)

Fenugreek, with its multifaceted nature as a culinary spice and herbal remedy, resonates through the ages as a symbol of nourishment and well-being.

Uses

Topical Applications

- **Skin health**: Fenugreek seeds or oil are used topically for skin health. Their anti-inflammatory properties may soothe irritated skin and alleviate conditions like eczema.
- **Hair care**: Fenugreek is often used in hair masks or oils to promote hair growth and address issues like dandruff.

Oral Consumption

- **Digestive aid**: Fenugreek has a long history of use as a digestive aid. Consuming fenugreek seeds or supplements may help alleviate indigestion and promote healthy digestion.
- **Lactation support**: Fenugreek is popular among nursing mothers, as it is believed to support lactation. It is often consumed in the form of teas or capsules.

Properties

- **Galactagogue**: Fenugreek is renowned for its galactagogue properties, potentially increasing milk production in lactating women.
- **Anti-inflammatory and antioxidant**: The herb exhibits anti-inflammatory and antioxidant properties contributing to its potential benefits for skin health and overall well-being.
- **Blood sugar regulation**: Fenugreek may help regulate blood sugar levels, thereby making it of interest for individuals with diabetes or those aiming to manage blood glucose.

History and Cultural Significance

Fenugreek has ancient roots in Ayurveda and traditional Chinese medicine where it was used for various health purposes including digestive support and respiratory health.

Egyptian and Greek civilizations also recognized fenugreek's medicinal properties.

Fenugreek holds cultural and historical significance in Islam. It is mentioned in Islamic traditions for its medicinal properties and has been traditionally used for various health purposes.

Feverfew (*Tanacetum parthenium*)

Feverfew supplements, capsules, and teas are readily available for those seeking natural approaches to migraine prevention. It is often included in herbal blends targeting headache relief.

Uses

Topical Applications

- **Migraine relief**: Feverfew is sometimes used topically —with crushed leaves applied to the skin—for its potential to alleviate migraines and headaches.
- **Skin conditions**: Some traditional practices involve using feverfew for skin conditions such as dermatitis and psoriasis due to its anti-inflammatory properties.

Oral Consumption

- **Migraine prevention**: Feverfew gained fame for its use in preventing migraines. Consuming feverfew supplements or fresh leaves is believed to reduce the frequency and severity of migraines.
- **Arthritis support**: It has been traditionally used for arthritis with proponents suggesting that its anti-inflammatory properties may offer relief.

Properties

- **Anti-inflammatory and analgesic**: Feverfew is known for its anti-inflammatory and analgesic properties, which contribute to its potential in relieving pain and discomfort.
- **Parthenolide content**: Parthenolide—a compound found in feverfew—is believed to play a role in its therapeutic effects, particularly in migraine prevention.

History and Cultural Significance

Feverfew has roots in ancient Greek and Roman traditions where it was used for various ailments including fevers—hence its name—and inflammation. It was recognized for its medicinal properties by herbalists such as Dioscorides and Pliny.

In European folklore, feverfew was considered a protective herb. It was often planted around homes to ward off illnesses and evil spirits. The herb was later introduced to England where it gained popularity in traditional herbalism.

Flaxseed (*Linum usitatissimum*)

Flaxseed supplements including flaxseed oil capsules and ground flaxseed are popular for people seeking to enhance their omega-3 intake and overall nutrition.

Uses

Topical Applications

- **Skin health**: Flaxseed oil, rich in omega-3 fatty acids, is used topically for its moisturizing properties. It may help soothe dry skin and alleviate conditions like eczema and psoriasis.
- **Hair care**: Flaxseed oil is incorporated into hair masks or applied directly to promote hair health, thus, providing nourishment to the scalp and strands.

Oral Consumption

- **Digestive health**: Ground flaxseeds are often consumed for their soluble fiber content, subsequently aiding in digestive health and promoting regular bowel movements.
- **Heart health**: Flaxseed's omega-3 fatty acids may contribute to heart health by reducing inflammation and supporting healthy cholesterol levels.

Properties

- **Omega-3 fatty acids**: Flaxseed is a rich source of alpha-linolenic acid (ALA), an omega-3 fatty acid. ALA has anti-inflammatory properties and is crucial for overall well-being.
- **Dietary fiber**: Flaxseeds contain both soluble and insoluble fiber supporting digestive health and providing a sense of fullness.
- **Lignans**: Flaxseeds are a primary source of lignans, which have antioxidant properties and may contribute to hormonal balance.

History and Cultural Significance

Flax has a long history of cultivation and use, dating back to ancient civilizations such as Mesopotamia and Egypt. It was valued for its versatile properties, including its fibers for textiles and its seeds for nutrition. Ancient Greeks and Romans also recognized the health benefits of flaxseeds.

In traditional European herbalism, flaxseed was used for respiratory issues, digestive complaints, and skin conditions.

In TCM, flaxseed was employed for its cooling properties, believed to balance the body's internal heat.

Garcinia Cambogia (*Garcinia gummi-gutta*)

Garcinia cambogia remains a notable player in the weight management industry with supplements widely available for those exploring natural approaches to weight loss.

Uses

Topical Applications

Garcinia cambogia is primarily consumed orally and its topical applications are limited. However, extracts or formulations containing its active compound—hydroxycitric acid (HCA)—are sometimes included in topical products for potential skin benefits.

Oral Consumption

- **Weight management**: Garcinia cambogia gained popularity for its potential role in weight management. It is often consumed in supplement form, as HCA is believed to inhibit an enzyme that helps the body store fat.
- **Appetite suppression**: Some users take garcinia cambogia supplements to potentially suppress appetite and reduce food intake.
- **Digestive health**: In traditional medicine, garcinia cambogia has been used for digestive issues due to promoting bowel regularity.

Properties

- **HCA**: The key active ingredient in garcinia cambogia is HCA. HCA is believed to block an enzyme called citrate lyase that the body uses to produce fat.
- **Appetite-suppressant**: Garcinia cambogia is thought to influence serotonin levels in the brain, potentially contributing to appetite suppression and improved mood.

- **Potential lipid-lowering effects**: Some studies suggest that garcinia cambogia may have lipid-lowering effects, consequently impacting cholesterol levels.

History and Cultural Significance

Garcinia cambogia has a history in traditional Ayurvedic medicine, where it was used for digestive issues and as a flavoring agent in culinary preparations.

In Ayurveda, the fruit rind which contains HCA is used for its therapeutic effects.

Garlic (*Allium sativum*)

Garlic gained recognition during World War I and II for its potential antiseptic properties. It was used to prevent infections and promote healing among wounded soldiers.

Uses

Topical Applications

- **Skin conditions**: Garlic has been used topically for various skin conditions due to its potential antibacterial and anti-inflammatory properties. It may be applied to wounds, acne, or fungal infections.
- **Wart removal**: Traditional remedies include using crushed garlic on warts for its purported antiviral effects.

Oral Consumption

- **Cardiovascular health**: Garlic is often consumed for its potential cardiovascular benefits. Allicin, a compound formed when garlic is crushed or chopped, is believed to contribute to improved heart health.

- **Immune support**: Garlic is valued for its immune-boosting properties. Regular consumption is thought to enhance the body's ability to fight infections.
- **Antimicrobial properties**: Garlic is known for its antimicrobial properties, potentially helping to combat bacterial, viral, and fungal infections.

Properties

- **Allicin and sulfur compounds**: Allicin, a sulfur compound in garlic, is responsible for its distinctive odor and is linked to many of its health benefits including its antimicrobial and cardiovascular effects.
- **Antioxidant content**: Garlic contains antioxidants that may help neutralize free radicals contributing to its potential role in reducing oxidative stress.
- **Anti-inflammatory effects**: Garlic is recognized for its anti-inflammatory effects, which may be beneficial for various conditions including arthritis and respiratory issues.

History and Cultural Significance

Garlic has an extensive history of use in ancient civilizations including Egyptian, Greek, and Roman cultures. It was used for medicinal purposes and even eaten by ancient athletes for strength. It also became a part of numerous traditional folk remedies for conditions ranging from infections to respiratory issues. It was used as a natural antibiotic.

In TCM, garlic was recommended for digestive health and its warming properties.

Ginger (*Zingiber officinale*)

Ginger played a pivotal role in the spice trade, subsequently becoming one of the most traded commodities between Asia and Europe during the Middle Ages.

Uses

Topical Applications

- **Pain relief**: Ginger has been used topically for pain relief, especially for conditions like arthritis and muscle soreness. Ginger oil or poultices may be applied to affected areas.
- **Nausea and headaches**: Some people find relief from nausea and headaches by inhaling the aroma of ginger essential oil.

Oral Consumption

- **Digestive aid**: Consuming ginger—whether in tea, capsules, or freshly grated—may help alleviate indigestion and nausea.
- **Anti-inflammatory effects**: Regular consumption of ginger is associated with anti-inflammatory effects contributing to joint and overall health.
- **Immune support**: Ginger is valued for its immune-boosting properties, potentially helping the body fend off infections.

Properties

- **Gingerol and bioactive compounds**: Gingerol is the main bioactive compound in ginger responsible for its distinctive flavor and many of its health benefits. It has potent antioxidant and anti-inflammatory effects.

- **Anti-nausea properties**: Ginger's anti-nausea effects make it a popular remedy for motion sickness, morning sickness during pregnancy, and nausea related to chemotherapy.
- **Antimicrobial effects**: Ginger has demonstrated antimicrobial properties potentially helping to combat certain infections.

History and Cultural Significance

Ginger has ancient roots in Chinese, Indian, and Middle Eastern medicine. It was highly prized for its medicinal properties including its warming effects and benefits for digestion. It was a common ingredient in various herbal formulations.

In Ayurveda, ginger was used to balance the body's doshas and enhance vitality.

In TCM, ginger was used to address conditions associated with cold and dampness such as joint pain and digestive issues.

Ginkgo (*Ginkgo biloba*)

Ginkgo biloba's journey from ancient Chinese medicine to global recognition reflects its enduring appeal and cultural significance.

Uses

Topical Applications

- **Skin health**: Ginkgo biloba extract—when used topically—is believed to have antioxidant properties that can benefit the skin. It may be included in skincare formulations for its potential to protect against oxidative stress.

- **Hair care**: Some hair products incorporate ginkgo biloba for its purported role in promoting hair health.

Oral Consumption

- **Cognitive support**: Ginkgo biloba is often consumed orally for cognitive support. It is believed to enhance memory and concentration, particularly in people experiencing mild cognitive impairment.
- **Peripheral circulation**: Ginkgo is used for promoting peripheral circulation, potentially benefiting conditions like intermittent claudication.
- **Antioxidant effects**: The antioxidant properties of ginkgo biloba are thought to contribute to its overall health benefits.

Properties

- **Flavonoids and terpenoids**: Ginkgo biloba contains flavonoids and terpenoids, which are believed to have antioxidant effects protecting cells from damage caused by free radicals.
- **Ginkgolides and bilobalide**: Ginkgo leaves contain unique compounds called ginkgolides and bilobalide, which may influence blood flow and have anti-inflammatory effects.
- **Neuroprotective potential**: Ginkgo is explored for its potential neuroprotective effects, which may be attributed to its ability to improve blood flow and reduce oxidative stress in the brain.

History and Cultural Significance

Ginkgo biloba has a deep-rooted history in TCM where it was used for various ailments including respiratory issues and cognitive function. The ginkgo tree, known as the maidenhair tree, is revered and often planted near temples.

Ginkgo biloba became known in Europe in the 18th century, and it gained prominence as a medicinal herb in the 20th century. It was embraced for its potential to support cognitive function and overall well-being.

Notably, ginkgo trees were among the few living things to survive the atomic bomb in Hiroshima, hence, symbolizing resilience and endurance. The ginkgo tree has since become a symbol of hope and peace.

Goldenseal (*Hydrastis canadensis*)

Goldenseal is a staple in contemporary herbalism, especially in North America.

Uses

Topical Applications

- **Skin conditions**: Goldenseal is used topically for various skin conditions, such as eczema, rashes, and wounds. Its antimicrobial properties are believed to support healing.
- **Eye wash**: Infusions or solutions containing goldenseal have been used as an eyewash for conditions like conjunctivitis.

Oral Consumption

- **Immune support**: Goldenseal is often consumed orally for immune support with its active compounds believed to have antimicrobial effects.
- **Digestive health**: Traditionally, goldenseal has been used for digestive issues, including promoting healthy digestion and addressing symptoms of indigestion.

Properties

- **Berberine content**: Goldenseal contains berberine—a compound with recognized antimicrobial properties. Berberine is believed to be a key contributor to goldenseal's medicinal effects.
- **Anti-inflammatory effects**: Goldenseal is known for its anti-inflammatory properties, which may contribute to its use in addressing various conditions including respiratory issues.

History and Cultural Significance

Goldenseal has a rich history in the traditional medicine of Indigenous American tribes, particularly the Cherokee and Iroquois. It was used for various ailments, including skin conditions and digestive issues. They referred to goldenseal as "yellow root" and held it in high regard.

European settlers learned about goldenseal from the native Americans and adopted its use in their own herbal traditions. In 19th-century eclectic medicine in the United States, goldenseal was a valued remedy for a range of conditions including infections.

Due to overharvesting and habitat loss, goldenseal is considered at risk in the wild. This has led to conservation efforts to protect and sustain its populations.

Hawthorn (*Crataegus monogyna*)

Hawthorn is often included in formulations targeting heart health and is sometimes combined with other herbs known for cardiovascular benefits.

Uses

Topical Applications

- **Skin conditions**: While hawthorn is primarily known for internal use, some herbalists recommend topical applications for certain skin conditions. Infused oils or creams with hawthorn may be used.
- **Anti-inflammatory effects**: External use is less common, but hawthorn's anti-inflammatory properties might contribute to skin benefits.

Oral Consumption

- **Cardiovascular health**: Hawthorn is renowned for its cardiovascular benefits. It is often consumed orally to support heart health, enhance circulation, and manage conditions like high blood pressure.
- **Heart tonic**: Hawthorn is considered a heart tonic, and its consumption is associated with strengthening the cardiovascular system.
- **Digestive aid**: Traditionally, hawthorn has been used for digestive support addressing issues like indigestion.

Properties

- **Flavonoids and oligomeric proanthocyanidins**: Hawthorn contains flavonoids and oligomeric proanthocyanidins, which are believed to contribute to its cardiovascular effects by dilating blood vessels and improving blood flow.
- **Cardiotonic effects**: The cardiotonic effects of hawthorn are attributed to its ability to enhance the force of cardiac contractions, consequently supporting overall heart function.
- **Antioxidant content**: Hawthorn's antioxidant properties may help combat oxidative stress, thus, contributing to its overall health benefits.

History and Cultural Significance

Hawthorn has deep roots in traditional European herbal medicine. It was historically used to treat cardiovascular issues, therefore, earning it the nickname "heart herb." European herbalists have used various parts of the hawthorn plant including the berries, leaves, and flowers.

Hawthorn found its way into TCM where it was used to address conditions related to blood circulation, promote digestion, and alleviate food stagnation—a condition in which the contents of the stomach lingers for longer than usual often caused by over-consumption.

Hoodia (*Hoodia gordonii*)

Hoodia's journey begins with its use by the San people, but global recognition for its potential appetite-suppressant properties underscores the intersection of cultural wisdom and contemporary health trends.

Uses

Oral Consumption

- **Appetite suppression**: Hoodia gained popularity for its supposed appetite-suppressant properties. Traditionally, it was believed to help indigenous communities endure long hunts by reducing hunger.
- **Weight management**: Hoodia is often marketed as a natural weight management aid, with some formulations including it as an ingredient in dietary supplements.

Properties

- **P57 molecule**: Hoodia's appetite-suppressant effects are attributed to the presence of the P57 molecule. This molecule is believed to influence the hypothalamus, thus, sending signals of fullness to the brain.
- **Limited scientific evidence**: It is important to note that while hoodia's traditional use suggests potential benefits, scientific evidence supporting its efficacy for appetite suppression is limited and more research is needed.

History and Cultural Significance

Hoodia has a long history of use among the San people of Southern Africa, particularly in the Kalahari Desert. It was traditionally consumed by hunters to stave off hunger during extended journeys. The San people chewed on the hoodia plant to suppress appetite and thirst.

Hoodia gained international attention in the early 2000s when it was promoted as a natural appetite suppressant. The plant's potential weight-loss benefits led to its inclusion in various dietary supplements.

The surge in popularity raised concerns about sustainability and ethical sourcing, as overharvesting became a risk.

Horse Chestnut (*Aesculus hippocastanum*)

Horse chestnut is often integrated into holistic health approaches combining herbal remedies with lifestyle modifications for circulatory well-being.

Uses

Horse chestnut trees are commonly planted in urban landscapes for their aesthetic value and shade, but that is not where their usefulness ends.

Topical Applications

- **Venous concerns**: Horse chestnut is often used topically in creams or ointments for its potential to alleviate symptoms related to poor venous circulation. This includes conditions like varicose veins and swollen legs.
- **Anti-inflammatory effects**: The plant's anti-inflammatory properties may contribute to its topical use for soothing skin and addressing inflammation.

Oral Consumption

- **Venotonic effects**: Orally, horse chestnut is known for its venotonic effects i.e., it may help support and strengthen blood vessels.
- **Edema and swelling**: It is traditionally used for conditions associated with edema and swelling, especially those related to venous insufficiency.

- **Chronic venous insufficiency (CVI)**: Horse chestnut extracts are sometimes included in oral supplements targeting CVI, a condition where veins have difficulty returning blood to the heart.

Properties

- **Aescin content**: The active compound in horse chestnut is aescin believed to have anti-inflammatory and venotonic effects.
- **Anti-inflammatory effects**: Horse chestnut's anti-inflammatory properties may contribute to its ability to reduce swelling and improve circulation.

History and Cultural Significance

The use of horse chestnut has its origin in European herbalism where it has been historically used for circulatory issues. Folk medicine traditions often included the use of horse chestnut for addressing a range of ailments—from hemorrhoids to leg cramps.

It gained popularity in the 19th century as a remedy for various conditions related to venous circulation.

Kava (*Piper methysticum*)

Kava supplements are sometimes sought for stress and anxiety management, thus, leveraging its traditional reputation for relaxation.

Uses

Oral Consumption

Relaxation and anxiety: Kava is renowned for its relaxing effects. It is often used to treat anxiety, insomnia, and other neurotic disorders.

Properties

Kavalactones: The active compounds in kava are kavalactones, which interact with neurotransmitter receptors, hence, contributing to its calming effects.

Anxiolytic and relaxant effects: Kavalactones are thought to affect gamma-aminobutyric acid (GABA) receptors resulting in anxiolytic and muscle relaxant effects.

History and Cultural Significance

Kava has a rich history in the cultures of the Pacific Islands including Fiji, Vanuatu, Tonga, and Samoa. It is deeply ingrained in social, spiritual, and ceremonial practices. It plays a central role in various rituals including welcoming guests, resolving conflicts, and marking important life events.

Traditionally, kava ceremonies involve the preparation and consumption of the beverage, therefore, fostering a sense of unity and connection. The sharing of kava is often accompanied by rituals that emphasize respect and communal bonds.

Lavender (*Lavandula angustifolia*)

The modern popularity of lavender in aromatherapy has surged with its essential oil finding applications in relaxation and stress relief.

Uses

Topical Applications

- **Skin soothing**: Lavender is widely used topically for its skin-soothing properties. It may aid in alleviating minor burns, insect bites, and skin irritations.
- **Aromatherapy**: Essential oil derived from lavender is often used in aromatherapy for relaxation, stress reduction, and promoting sleep.

Oral Consumption

- **Calming infusions**: Lavender infusions—made by steeping dried lavender flowers—are consumed orally for their calming effects. They are popular choices for herbal teas.
- **Digestive aid**: Lavender has been historically used to address mild digestive discomfort, and its consumption may contribute to a sense of calm.

Properties

- **Linalool and linalyl acetate**: The key constituents of lavender such as linalool and linalyl acetate contribute to its calming and anti-inflammatory effects.
- **Relaxant and anti-inflammatory effects**: Lavender is recognized for its ability to induce relaxation, reduce stress, and potentially alleviate inflammation.

History and Cultural Significance

Lavender has a long history of use in ancient Mediterranean cultures where it was valued for its aromatic qualities and potential medicinal benefits.

The Romans, Greeks, and Egyptians used lavender in various applications including bathing, perfumery, and medicinal preparations.

Lavender continued to be popular in the Middle Ages and Renaissance where it was incorporated into potpourris, sachets, and herbal remedies.

Licorice Root (*Glycyrrhiza glabra*)

Licorice is included in some herbal formulations aimed at supporting respiratory health, especially in products addressing occasional coughs and throat irritation.

Uses

Oral Consumption

- **Gastrointestinal support**: Licorice root has been historically used to support digestive health. It may help soothe the digestive tract and address mild discomfort.
- **Respiratory health**: In traditional medicine, licorice has been included in formulations to address respiratory issues and promote a healthy respiratory system.

Properties

- **Glycyrrhizin content**: The primary active compound in licorice root is glycyrrhizin, which imparts the characteristic sweet taste and contributes to its potential health benefits.
- **Anti-inflammatory and antioxidant effects**: Licorice root is recognized for its anti-inflammatory and antioxidant properties, which may contribute to its traditional uses in promoting wellness.

History and Cultural Significance

Licorice has a rich history dating back to ancient civilizations such as Mesopotamia where it was valued for its sweetness and potential medicinal properties.

Licorice root was used by ancient Egyptians for its sweetness in confections and beverages. It was also believed to have health-promoting qualities.

In ancient Greece, it was employed for its potential soothing effects on the respiratory and digestive systems.

It found its way into various traditional medicine systems including Ayurveda and TCM.

Milk Thistle (*Silybum marianum*)

Milk thistle's distinctive appearance with its spiky purple flower head and milky sap contributed to its recognition as a herb of great importance.

Uses

Oral Consumption

- **Liver support**: Milk thistle has hepatoprotective properties and is commonly used to support liver health, especially in conditions associated with liver damage or inflammation.
- **Detoxification**: Traditionally, milk thistle has been associated with detoxification and helping the liver process toxins more efficiently.

Properties

Silymarin content: The key active component in milk thistle is silymarin—a complex of flavonoids with antioxidant and anti-inflammatory properties.

Hepatoprotective and antioxidant effects: Silymarin is recognized for its hepatoprotective effects by shielding liver cells from damage. Additionally, its antioxidant properties contribute to overall cellular health.

History and Cultural Significance

Milk thistle has historical roots in Mediterranean cultures where it was valued for its medicinal properties. Ancient herbalists noted its potential benefits for liver-related ailments.

Throughout traditional herbalism, milk thistle was employed to address various liver disorders including jaundice and hepatitis.

Mugwort (*Artemisia vulgaris*)

Mugwort is associated with dreamwork and divination. In some cultures, it is believed to enhance dream recall and facilitate vivid dreams.

Uses

Topical Applications

- **Skin conditions**: Mugwort has been used topically to address various skin conditions. Its anti-inflammatory and soothing properties make it a candidate for treating minor irritations and skin discomfort.
- **Aromatherapy**: Mugwort leaves are sometimes used in aromatherapy practices when dried, subsequently

providing a fragrant experience believed to induce relaxation.

Oral Consumption

- **Digestive support**: Traditionally, mugwort has been consumed orally to support digestive health. It is thought to have mild carminative effects that help alleviate digestive discomfort.
- **Culinary uses**: In some cultures, mugwort leaves are used in cooking and are added to dishes for their unique flavor.

Properties

- **Artemisinin content**: One of the notable compounds in mugwort is artemisinin known for its potential antimalarial properties.
- **Anti-inflammatory and antispasmodic effects**: Mugwort is recognized for its anti-inflammatory and antispasmodic effects, which contribute to its traditional uses in addressing various conditions.

History and Cultural Significance

In TCM, mugwort is known as "Ai Ye" and is used in moxibustion—a therapy involving the burning of mugwort to stimulate acupoints.

Mugwort holds cultural significance in folklore and rituals. In European traditions, it was believed to offer protection against evil spirits and was used in rituals to ward off negativity. Native American tribes such as the Cherokee used mugwort in ceremonies and believed it had spiritual properties.

Passionflower (*Passiflora incarnata*)

Passionflower's unique floral structure led to its association with Christian symbolism, especially with the elements in the story of *The Passion of* the Christ. The tendrils were thought to represent the whips used in the flagellation and the central flower column was associated with the cross.

Uses

Topical Applications

- **Limited topical use**: Passionflower is primarily used for oral consumption and its topical applications are limited. Its focus lies in internal use for its calming properties.
- **Soothing compresses**: In some instances, passionflower may be used in herbal compresses to soothe minor skin irritations.

Oral Consumption

- **Calming infusions**: Passionflower is often consumed orally in the form of teas or infusions for its calming and relaxing effects. It is known to promote a sense of tranquility.
- **Supplements**: Passionflower supplements including capsules and tinctures are used to harness its potential benefits for mental well-being.

Properties

- **Alkaloids and flavonoids**: Passionflower contains various compounds including alkaloids and flavonoids.

These constituents contribute to its soothing and calming properties.

- **Anxiolytic and sedative effects**: Passionflower is recognized for its anxiolytic (anxiety-reducing) and sedative effects. It promotes relaxation and helps alleviate symptoms of stress.

History and Cultural Significance

Native American tribes—particularly those in the southeastern United States—historically used passionflower for its calming effects. The Cherokee particularly valued it for its potential to soothe nervousness.

In the 17th century, European colonists learned about passion-flower from Native American communities. It was later adopted into European herbal traditions where it became known for its calming properties.

Peppermint (*Mentha * piperita*)

Traditional herbalists value peppermint for its ability to soothe digestive issues, alleviate headaches, and provide a sense of invigoration.

Uses

Topical Applications

- **Cooling compresses**: Peppermint's menthol content makes it suitable for topical applications. It is used in cooling compresses to soothe minor skin irritations and provide relief.
- **Aromatherapy**: Peppermint essential oil is popular in aromatherapy believed to invigorate the senses and promote mental clarity.

Oral Consumption

- **Digestive aid**: Peppermint is renowned for its digestive benefits. Consumed as a tea or added to culinary dishes, it can help alleviate symptoms of indigestion and promote digestive comfort.
- **Respiratory support**: Peppermint tea or inhalation of its aroma is often used for respiratory support, consequently providing a refreshing sensation.

Properties

Menthol content: The key active component in peppermint is menthol. This compound contributes to peppermint's characteristic cooling sensation and various therapeutic properties.

Antispasmodic and analgesic effects: Peppermint is recognized for its antispasmodic effects, which make it valuable in addressing digestive spasms. It also possesses analgesic properties contributing to its use for minor pain relief.

History and Cultural Significance

Peppermint has a history dating back to ancient civilizations. It was used in ancient Egypt and Rome for its refreshing aroma and medicinal properties.

Romans used peppermint as a flavoring agent and it was considered a symbol of hospitality. It found a place in European herbal traditions where it was cultivated in monastery gardens.

Pomegranate (*Punica granatum*)

Pomegranate features prominently in Middle Eastern and Mediterranean cuisines. Its juicy arils are used in salads, desserts, and beverages adding a burst of flavor and nutritional richness.

Uses

Topical Applications

- **Skin care**: Pomegranate oil and extracts are used topically in skincare products. Its antioxidant properties may contribute to skin health potentially aiding in reducing signs of aging and promoting a radiant complexion.
- **Wound healing**: Traditional uses include applying pomegranate to wounds for its potential wound-healing properties.

Oral Consumption

- **Antioxidant boost**: Consuming pomegranate whether as whole fruit or juice provides a rich source of antioxidants, which may contribute to overall health.
- **Cardiovascular support**: Pomegranate is associated with cardiovascular benefits including potential effects on cholesterol levels and blood pressure.

Properties

- **Antioxidant rich**: Pomegranate is rich in antioxidants including polyphenols and anthocyanins. These compounds contribute to its potential health-promoting effects.
- **Anti-inflammatory effects**: Studies suggest that pomegranate may possess anti-inflammatory properties, which could be beneficial in addressing inflammatory conditions.

History and Cultural Significance

Pomegranate has a storied history often symbolizing fertility, abundance, and prosperity in ancient civilizations. It was revered in Greek, Roman, and Egyptian cultures. In Ayurveda, it is used for its digestive and cardiovascular benefits.

In ancient Persia, the fruit was associated with immortality, and its consumption was believed to confer health benefits. Traditional Persian medicine valued pomegranate for its cooling properties and as a remedy for digestive issues.

Red Clover (*Trifolium pratense*)

Red clover supplements and teas are popular natural alternatives for managing menopausal symptoms providing women with potential relief.

Uses

Topical Applications

- **Skin conditions**: Red clover is sometimes used topically to address skin conditions due to its anti-inflammatory properties. It may be included in creams or ointments for its potential soothing effects.
- **Wound healing**: Traditionally, red clover has been applied to wounds to aid in the healing process.

Oral Consumption

- **Menopausal symptoms**: Red clover is commonly consumed orally as an herbal remedy for menopausal symptoms. It contains compounds known as isoflavones that may have estrogen-like effects.

- **Blood purification**: Traditionally, red clover has been used as a blood purifier believed to support overall health by promoting detoxification.

Properties

- **Isoflavones**: Red clover is a rich source of isoflavones including genistein and daidzein. These compounds are phytoestrogens, hence, may influence hormonal balance.
- **Nutrient content**: The plant contains essential nutrients such as vitamins, minerals, and antioxidants contributing to its potential health-promoting properties.

History and Cultural Significance

Red clover has roots in traditional medicine practices where it was valued for its potential as a blood purifier and for addressing various ailments.

In Celtic folklore, red clover was considered a symbol of protection and was believed to ward off evil spirits. Native American tribes used red clover for medicinal purposes including respiratory support and skin conditions.

Rhodiola (*Rhodiola rosea*)

As stress continues to be a prevalent concern in contemporary life, Rhodiola remains relevant for people seeking natural approaches to stress management and overall well-being.

Uses

Topical Applications

Adaptogenic properties: While not commonly used topically, Rhodiola's adaptogenic properties, which help the body cope with stress, may indirectly contribute to skin health. Stress management is a key factor in maintaining overall skin well-being.

Oral Consumption

- **Stress and fatigue relief**: Rhodiola is primarily consumed orally for its adaptogenic effects. It is recognized for its potential to combat stress, alleviate fatigue, and enhance overall resilience.
- **Cognitive support**: Some users take rhodiola for cognitive support believing it may improve mental clarity, concentration, and memory.

Properties

- **Adaptogenic compounds**: Rhodiola contains adaptogenic compounds including rosavin and salidroside that are believed to contribute to its stress-relieving effects.
- **Antioxidant activity**: The herb possesses antioxidant properties, therefore, helps combat oxidative stress and supports cellular health.

History and Cultural Significance

Rhodiola has a rich history in traditional medicine, particularly in Siberian and Scandinavian cultures. It was used to combat the harsh effects of the cold climate, increase stamina, and cope with stress.

Scandinavian cultures consideredinging it a tonic for resilience in the face of challenging conditions and used Rhodiola to make herbal teas.

Traditional healers valued rhodiola for its potential to enhance physical and mental endurance. In Siberian folklore, Rhodiola was often referred to as the "golden root" and was believed to bestow strength and vitality upon those who consumed it.

Sage (*Salvia officinalis*)

Its name is derived from the Latin word "salvere" and means "to save" or "to heal," thus, underscoring its healing properties.

Uses

Topical Applications

- **Antiseptic and anti-inflammatory**: Sage's antiseptic and anti-inflammatory properties make it suitable for topical applications. It has been used in salves or infused oils to address minor skin irritations and promote wound healing.
- **Oral health**: Sage-infused mouthwashes or gargles are employed for their potential antibacterial properties, thereby contributing to oral health.

Oral Consumption

- **Digestive aid**: Sage has a history of use as a digestive aid. Consuming sage tea or incorporating sage into meals may help alleviate digestive discomfort.
- **Menopausal support**: Sage is recognized for its potential to manage menopausal symptoms, particularly

hot flashes. It contains compounds that may influence hormonal balance.

Properties

- **Essential oils**: Sage contains essential oils including thujone and camphor which contribute to its aromatic and medicinal properties.
- **Antioxidant and anti-inflammatory effects**: The herb possesses antioxidant compounds, hence, offers protection against oxidative stress. Its anti-inflammatory effects may contribute to its traditional uses.

History and Cultural Significance

Sage has a venerable history rooted in ancient civilizations such as Greece and Rome. It was valued for its medicinal properties and often associated with wisdom and longevity.

Ancient Roman physicians recommended sage for its potential to address various ailments including digestive issues.

Sage has been a staple in traditional medicine across cultures. In Ayurveda, it was used for its potential digestive benefits, and Native American tribes employed it for various health purposes.

Saw Palmetto (*Serenoa repens*)

This fan palm can grow 2–10 ft tall and is prized for its nutritious berries.

Uses

Topical Applications

- **Hair health**: Some people use saw palmetto topically in hair products believing it may promote hair health. Its potential impact on hormonal balance is thought to contribute to this effect.
- **Skin care**: Saw palmetto's anti-inflammatory properties may be beneficial in skincare, potentially addressing conditions like acne or irritation.

Oral Consumption

- **Prostate health**: One of the most common uses of saw palmetto is for prostate health. It is often consumed as an oral supplement to alleviate symptoms of benign prostatic hyperplasia (BPH).
- **Hormonal balance**: Saw palmetto is believed to have an impact on hormonal balance, making it a potential remedy for conditions influenced by hormones such as PCOS.

Properties

- **Fatty acids and phytosterols**: Saw palmetto contains fatty acids and phytosterols believed to contribute to its potential anti-inflammatory and hormonal-modulating properties.
- **Anti-inflammatory effects**: The herb exhibits anti-inflammatory effects that may be beneficial in addressing conditions related to inflammation.

History and Cultural Significance

Native American tribes, particularly the Seminole and Miccosukee, historically used saw palmetto berries as a food source and traditional medicine. Indigenous communities valued the plant for its potential to address various health concerns including reproductive and urinary issues.

Early American settlers learned about saw palmetto from indigenous communities, subsequently incorporating it into their own folk medicine practices.

Saw palmetto has a history of use in traditional medicine where it was employed for its potential diuretic, expectorant, and nutritive properties.

Soy (*Glycine max*)

Soy provides a sustainable protein source and essential nutrients for balanced nutrition and is a key player in contemporary plant-based diets. Its nutritional density makes it a valuable source of protein for people adopting vegetarian or vegan lifestyles.

Uses

Topical Applications

Skin care: Soy is rich in compounds like isoflavones and vitamin E making it a popular ingredient in skincare products. It is believed to contribute to skin health by providing antioxidant and moisturizing effects.

Oral Consumption

- **Nutritional support**: Soy is consumed orally for its nutritional profile. It is a source of protein, essential amino acids, and various vitamins and minerals.

- **Menopausal symptom relief**: Soy contains phytoestrogens and some people use soy products to alleviate menopausal symptoms, as these compounds may have estrogen-like effects.

Properties

- **Anti-aging properties**: Some topical formulations use soy for its potential anti-aging properties aiming to reduce the appearance of fine lines and wrinkles.
- **Isoflavones**: Soy is rich in isoflavones including genistein and daidzein, thus, influence hormonal balance.
- **Nutrient density**: Soy is nutritionally dense containing essential nutrients such as protein, fiber, vitamins (B-complex), and minerals (iron, calcium).

History and Cultural Significance

Soy has a long history of cultivation in East Asia, particularly in China. It was a staple in the diet used for its nutritional value and versatility. Ancient Chinese texts document the cultivation and consumption of soybeans recognizing their significance in traditional agriculture and cuisine.

Traditional Chinese medicine recognized the potential health benefits of soy, incorporating it into formulations to support overall well-being. Soy has immense cultural significance in East Asian cuisines, serving as a foundational ingredient in dishes like tofu, miso, and soy milk.

St John's Wort (*Hypericum perforatum*)

The plant's vibrant yellow flowers blooming around the summer solstice contribute to its association with light, warmth, and positive energy.

Uses

Topical Applications

- **Skin health**: St. John's Wort has been traditionally used topically for its potential benefits to the skin. It is believed to have anti-inflammatory and wound-healing properties making it suitable for addressing minor skin irritations.
- **Neuralgia and nerve pain**: Some people use St. John's Wort oil topically to alleviate nerve pain and symptoms of conditions like neuralgia.

Oral Consumption

- **Mood support**: St. John's Wort is commonly used orally to support mood and emotional well-being. It contains compounds such as hypericin and hyperforin that may influence neurotransmitter levels.
- **Mild to moderate depression**: It is often considered a natural remedy for mild to moderate depression; users subsequently seek its potential antidepressant effects.

Properties

- **Hypericin and hyperforin**: St. John's Wort contains hypericin and hyperforin believed to contribute to its mood-enhancing properties.

- **Antioxidant and anti-inflammatory effects**: The herb exhibits antioxidant and anti-inflammatory effects supporting its traditional use for skin conditions and overall health.

History and Cultural Significance

St. John's Wort has a rich history dating back to ancient civilizations where it was utilized for various medicinal purposes. Ancient Greek physicians including Hippocrates recognized its therapeutic potential and recommended it for its medicinal properties.

The plant's name is associated with the Christian feast of St. John the Baptist symbolizing its flowering around that time. In European folklore, it was believed to possess protective qualities and was associated with warding off evil spirits.

Tea Tree (*Melaleuca alternifolia*)

Tea tree oil—with its aromatic leaves—stands as a guardian in the realm of herbal remedies.

Uses

Topical Applications

- **Antiseptic and antibacterial**: Tea tree oil is renowned for its potent antiseptic and antibacterial properties. It is applied topically to treat cuts, wounds, acne, and various skin infections.
- **Skin conditions**: People use tea tree oil to alleviate conditions like psoriasis and eczema due to its anti-inflammatory effects.
- **Diluted for safety**: It is crucial to dilute tea tree oil before topical application to prevent skin irritation.

Oral Consumption

Tea tree oil-infused oral products, such as toothpaste and mouth-wash, are used for their potential benefits in promoting oral health. Its antimicrobial properties may contribute to combating bacteria in the mouth.

Properties

- **Terpenes and terpinen-4-ol**: Tea tree oil's active compounds including terpenes and terpinen-4-ol impart their antimicrobial and anti-inflammatory properties.
- **Antifungal and antiviral effects**: The oil exhibits antifungal and antiviral effects, making it valuable in addressing fungal infections and viral skin conditions.

History and Cultural Significance

Indigenous Australian communities, particularly the Bundjalung people, have a long history of using tea tree leaves for medicinal purposes. The leaves were crushed and applied to the skin to treat wounds and infections.

Captain James Cook's crew reportedly used tea tree leaves as a substitute for tea leading to the plant's name.

Tea tree oil regained recognition during World War II when it was included in soldiers' first aid kits. Its effectiveness in preventing infections contributed to its rediscovery and wide-spread use. After the war, tea tree oil production increased and it found its way into various skincare and medicinal applications.

Thunder God Vine (*Tripterygium wilfordii*)

Thunder god vine continues to be a subject of research, with ongoing clinical trials exploring its potential in treating autoimmune conditions and inflammatory disorders.

Uses

Topical Applications

- **Inflammatory conditions**: Thunder god vine has been traditionally used topically to address inflammatory skin conditions such as psoriasis and rheumatoid arthritis. Creams and ointments containing extracts from the plant are applied to affected areas.
- **Joint pain**: Some people use topical formulations to alleviate joint pain associated with arthritis.

Oral Consumption

- **Rheumatoid arthritis**: Thunder god vine is often taken orally as a potential treatment for rheumatoid arthritis. Some studies suggest that compounds in the plant may have anti-inflammatory effects.
- **Immune modulation**: Compounds in thunder god vine may modulate the immune system, making it a subject of interest in autoimmune conditions.

Properties

- **Triterpenoids**: Thunder god vine contains triterpenoids including triptolide and celastrol which are believed to contribute to their anti-inflammatory and immunosuppressive properties.
- **Immunosuppressive effects**: The plant exhibits immunosuppressive effects making it a subject of research for autoimmune conditions.

History and Cultural Significance

Thunder god vine has a long history in TCM where it has been used for centuries to address various health issues. It has been used for its potential to alleviate conditions related to inflammation, pain, and immune system imbalances. The use of thunder god vine for rheumatoid arthritis gained attention in the mid-20th century in China. It was recognized for its potential to reduce joint inflammation and pain.

Turmeric (*Curcuma longa*)

Uses

Turmeric has gained superfood status globally. Its use has expanded beyond traditional cuisines with people incorporating it into smoothies, lattes, and health-focused recipes.

Topical Applications

- **Skin anti-inflammatory agent**: Turmeric—with its active compound curcumin—is used topically for its anti-inflammatory properties. It may help soothe skin conditions like psoriasis, eczema, and acne.
- **Wound healing**: Turmeric paste is applied to wounds and cuts for its potential antiseptic and wound-healing effects.

Oral Consumption

- **Anti-inflammatory and antioxidant**: Turmeric is widely consumed orally for its anti-inflammatory and antioxidant properties. It is used in curries, teas, and golden milk to promote overall health.

- **Digestive aid**: Turmeric has a well-documented past of use as a digestive aid. It may help alleviate digestive issues and discomfort.

Properties

- **Curcumin**: Curcumin—the main active compound in turmeric—is known for its anti-inflammatory, antioxidant, and potential anticancer properties.
- **Antioxidant effects**: Turmeric exhibits potent antioxidant effects by scavenging free radicals and supporting cellular health.

History and Cultural Significance

Turmeric holds a revered place in Ayurveda—the traditional medicine of India. It is classified as a "Rasaayana" or rejuvenating herb used to balance doshas and promote overall health. Ayurvedic texts document turmeric's use for various conditions including respiratory and digestive issues.

In Indian culture, turmeric holds cultural and ritualistic significance. Turmeric paste—symbolizing purity and prosperity—is applied to the skin of the bride and groom in pre-wedding ceremonies.

Valerian (*Valeriana officinalis*)

Valerian is woven into herbal traditions across cultures. Its inclusion in herbal formulations reflects its enduring role as a gentle remedy for nervous system support and calming the restless mind.

Uses

Topical Applications

Relaxation and calming: Valerian—when used topically—is often in the form of essential oil. Its calming properties may be harnessed through aromatherapy or diluted oil application on pulse points for relaxation.

Oral Consumption

- **Sleep aid**: Valerian is primarily known for its potential as a natural sleep aid. It is often consumed orally in the form of tea, capsules, or tinctures to promote relaxation and improve sleep quality.
- **Anxiety and stress**: Some people use valerian for its anxiolytic effects that alleviate symptoms of anxiety and stress.

Properties

- **Valerenic acid**: Valerian contains valerenic acid—a compound believed to contribute to its sedative and anxiolytic effects.
- **Sedative and relaxant effects**: Valerian is recognized for its sedative and muscle relaxant properties, thus, making it a popular choice for those seeking natural remedies for sleep and relaxation.

History and Cultural Significance

Valerian's use can be traced back to ancient Greece and Rome. It was embraced for its potential to soothe nerves, ease tension, and induce restful sleep. The Greek physician Hippocrates and the Roman naturalist Pliny the Elder documented valerian's calming effects in their writings.

Valerian continued to be a staple in European herbal medicine during the Middle Ages and the Renaissance. It was often used as a remedy for nervous disorders and insomnia. Its reputation as a tranquilizer persisted leading to its inclusion in various herbal formulations.

White Mulberry Leaf (*Morus alba*)

White mulberry leaf and bark weave a narrative of vitality and balance with their storied history and cultural significance.

Uses

Topical Applications

- **Skin conditions**: White mulberry leaf extracts may be used topically to address certain skin conditions. The anti-inflammatory characteristics could potentially provide relief to irritated skin and diminish redness.
- **Cosmetic formulations**: In some skincare products, white mulberry leaf extracts are incorporated for their potential benefits in promoting even skin tone.

Oral Consumption

- **Blood sugar management**: White mulberry leaf is often consumed orally for its potential to help manage blood sugar levels. This is particularly relevant for individuals dealing with diabetes or those aiming to regulate glucose.
- **Antioxidant support**: The oral consumption of white mulberry leaf may provide antioxidant support resulting in overall well-being.

Properties

- **Polyphenols and flavonoids**: White mulberry leaf contains polyphenols and flavonoids, which are associated with antioxidant and anti-inflammatory effects.
- **Blood sugar regulation**: Compounds like 1-deoxynojirimycin (DNJ) in white mulberry leaf are thought to inhibit the breakdown of sugars, potentially contributing to blood sugar regulation.

History and Cultural Significance

In TCM, various parts of the white mulberry tree including the leaves and bark have been used for centuries. They were historically used for their potential to balance blood sugar. The plant's use aligns with the principles of balancing energy and promoting overall health in TCM.

White mulberry trees are historically significant due to their role in the silk industry. Mulberry leaves are the primary food source for silkworms contributing to the production of silk. The cultural and economic importance of white mulberry trees is intertwined with the silk trade's historical significance.

Yohimbe (*Pausinystalia johimbe*)

Yohimbe has a reputation as an aphrodisiac contributing to its association with vitality and sexual health.

Uses

Topical applications

Traditional rituals: Yohimbe bark has been used topically in some traditional African practices. The bark's alkaloids, particularly yohimbine, are believed to have stimulating effects and are sometimes applied in ceremonial rituals.

Oral Consumption

- **Aphrodisiac traditions**: Yohimbe is often consumed orally for its potential aphrodisiac properties. It is traditionally associated with enhancing sexual vitality and addressing certain aspects of sexual dysfunction.
- **Energy and stamina**: Some people use yohimbe as a natural energy booster relying on its stimulant properties to increase stamina and vitality.

Properties

- **Yohimbine alkaloids**: Yohimbe contains yohimbine and related alkaloids. Yohimbine is known for its vasodilatory effects, consequently increasing blood flow, and is sometimes explored for its role in sexual health.
- **Central nervous system stimulant**: Yohimbe is considered a central nervous system stimulant, and its properties are believed to contribute to increased alertness and energy.

History and Cultural Significance

Yohimbe has roots in traditional African medicine where it was historically used for various purposes including as a stimulant and aphrodisiac. Indigenous communities valued the bark for its potential to address certain health concerns.

Yohimbe gained attention in Western herbalism for its potential aphrodisiac effects. In the late 19th and early 20th centuries, it was explored in Western herbal practices as a remedy for sexual issues.

Chapter 6

Crafting Herbal Preparations

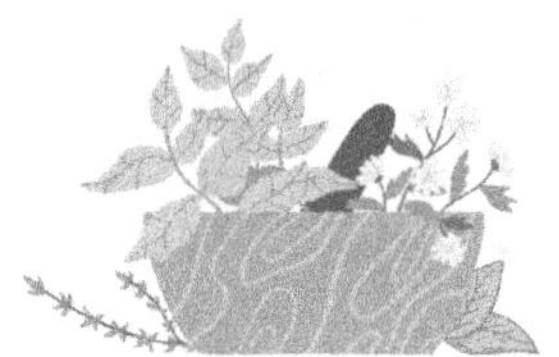

The Art of Brewing Herbal Teas

The art of brewing herbal teas is a delightful and versatile practice that spans cultures and centuries. Herbal teas, also known as tisanes, are caffeine-free infusions made from various plant materials like leaves, flowers, seeds, and roots. Here is how to brew herbal teas to create flavorsome, aromatic, and healthful beverages.

Choosing Quality Herbs

Selecting Fresh or Dried Herbs

Choose high-quality, organic herbs for optimal potency and purity. Depending on the intended use, select herbs with specific medicinal properties. Fresh herbs can be harvested from your garden or bought from a reliable source. Dried herbs should be of high quality, aromatic, and free from contaminants.

Single Herbs or Blends

If you are new to herbal teas, it is best to first experiment with one herb at a time. This will give you an idea of how the herbs taste individually and which ones may taste good together. Custom blends can include two or more different herbs for unique flavor profiles and potentially compound health benefits.

Equipment Needed

- **Tea Infuser or strainer**: For loose herbs, use a tea infuser or strainer to contain the plant material during brewing. Choose an infuser with enough space to accommodate the herb's expansion in water and to allow its flavors to release fully.
- **Teapot or teacup**: Brew larger quantities in a teapot or enjoy a single cup of your favorite herbal tea. Opt for teapots made of ceramic or clay to maintain a high temperature while the tea is steeping.
- **Kettle or water heater**: Boil water separately using a kettle or water heater when making an infusion, or add herbs to the water before boiling to make a decoction. Ensure the water quality is suitable for tea preparation.

Water Temperature

Boiling Water for Most Herbs

Bring water to a rolling boil and let it cool slightly before pouring over most herbs. Delicate herbs like chamomile or hibiscus may require slightly cooler water.

Different Temperatures for Different Herbs

Some herbs like green tea or peppermint may require specific water temperatures for optimal flavor extraction. Follow the recommended temperature guidelines for each herb.

Herb-to-Water Ratio

General Guidelines

Use about one to two teaspoons of dried herbs or one to two tablespoons of fresh herbs per cup. Adjust the ratio based on your personal preference or for stronger remedies.

Experiment with Ratios

Depending on the herb, you may need to experiment with ratios or blends with other herbs to find the perfect balance of flavor.

Sweeteners and Enhancements

Natural Sweeteners

Adjust sweetness to taste using honey, maple syrup, or agave for natural sweetness.

Citrus or Spices

Enhance flavors with a slice of citrus, ginger, or spices like cinnamon or cloves. Experiment with different combinations to find your preferred mix.

Serving

Strain loose herbs or leave them in the pot or cup based on personal preference. Some herbal teas like chamomile are traditionally served with the herb left in.

Health Considerations

Be mindful of the medicinal properties of the herbs you are taking, and how they may interact with medications you are taking or other contraindications such as underlying health conditions and allergies, and consult a healthcare professional if necessary. Ensure that the herbs used are safe for consumption and have not been treated with harmful pesticides or chemicals.

Storage of Prepared Tea

If not consumed immediately, store brewed herbal tea in the refrigerator. Consume within a day or two for optimal freshness.

Infusions and Decoctions

Infusions and decoctions are two traditional methods of extracting the medicinal properties and flavor from herbs, spices, or other plant materials. These methods involve steeping or boiling plant matter in water to create an herbal infusion or decoction.

Infusions

Making an infusion involves steeping herbs in hot or cold water for a specific time to extract the medicinal properties of herbs. Infusions are often used for teas and herbal drinks and should be prepared immediately before consumption as they have a limited shelf-life. This method is ideal for delicate plant parts like leaves and flowers, and is ideal for preserving volatile compounds and subtle flavors.

How to make an infusion:

1. Pour hot water over fresh or dry herbs. For a cold infusion, simply add the herbs to cold water.
2. Cover the infusion while steeping to retain volatile oils.
3. Steep for an average of 5–10 minutes, but this can vary based on the herb. Adjust the steeping time for the desired potency. Hot infusions require less time to steep than cold infusions, which are generally left to steep for several hours or overnight. Stronger infusions may result from longer steeping times.

Note: Pay attention to the brew's taste during steeping to prevent bitterness. Some herbs can become bitter if steeped for too long.

Decoctions

Decoctions are made by boiling herbs in water to extract medicinal compounds. This results in a brew that is stronger than an infusion. Decocting is ideal for herbs with heat-stable constituents and tough plant parts like roots, seeds, or bark which may require higher heat for extracting medicinal compounds.

How to make a decoction:

1. Add fresh or dry herbs and bring the water to a low boil.
2. Simmer with the lid on for 15–30 minutes depending on the herb used and the potency required.
3. Remove the decoction from heat and allow it to cool.
4. Strain out the plant matter.

Introduction to Carrier Oils and Essential Oils

In the realms of aromatherapy and natural wellness, carrier oils and essential oils play integral roles each contributing unique qualities to the symphony of holistic well-being. These oils derived from various plants, seeds, and nuts have been cherished for centuries for their aromatic, therapeutic, and skincare properties. To understand the essence of carrier oils and essential oils, we will explore their distinct characteristics.

Carrier Oils

Carrier oils, also known as base or fixed oils, are derived from the fatty portions of plants such as seeds, nuts, or kernels. Unlike essential oils, carrier oils do not evaporate and possess a mild aroma. These oils serve as a vehicle for diluting essential oils ensuring their safe application and enhancing their absorption into the skin.

Characteristics

- **Nutrient-rich**: Carrier oils are laden with essential fatty acids, vitamins, and minerals providing nourishment and hydration to the skin. Common examples include jojoba, sweet almond, and coconut oil.
- **Mild aroma**: Carrier oils have a subtle scent, often characterized by a gentle, nutty, or slightly sweet aroma. This mild fragrance allows them to complement, rather than overpower, the more potent scents of essential oils.
- **Skincare allies**: Due to their moisturizing properties, carrier oils are widely used in skincare routines, thereby offering a natural alternative to commercial moisturizers that may cause allergies. They can be applied directly to the skin or used as a base for essential oil blends.
- **Dilution medium**: Carrier oils act as a medium to dilute highly concentrated and potent essential oils, hence, ensuring their safe and effective application in aromatherapy or massage.

Essential Oils

Essential oils are highly concentrated extracts derived from aromatic plants. The parts used may differ from species to species. Essential oils capture the essence of the plant and contain potent aromatic compounds that contribute to their therapeutic and aromatic qualities. These oils are revered for their diverse applications in aromatherapy, holistic healing, and as natural fragrance agents.

Characteristics

- **Potent aromas**: Essential oils boast intense and captivating scents ranging from floral and citrusy to woody and earthy. These potent aromas form the foundation of aromatherapy, therefore, influencing mood, relaxation, and overall well-being.
- **Therapeutic properties**: Essential oils exhibit a spectrum of therapeutic properties including antimicrobial, anti-inflammatory, and stress-relieving attributes. Each essential oil carries a unique set of benefits making them versatile tools in holistic health practices.
- **Application methods**: Essential oils can be diffused into the air, applied topically—when appropriately diluted—or added to bathwater for aromatherapeutic benefits. The inhalation or topical application of essential oils facilitates their absorption into the bloodstream, consequently influencing physiological and psychological responses.
- **Distinct profiles**: Each essential oil has a distinct profile reflecting the plant's chemical composition. For instance, lavender oil is renowned for its calming properties, while peppermint oil is invigorating and refreshing.

Harmony in Practice

- **Synergistic relationship**: The synergy between carrier oils and essential oils is fundamental in aromatherapy. Carrier oils provide a gentle medium for diluting essential oils making them safer to apply and speeding up safe application while enhancing absorption into the skin.

- **Blending techniques**: Creating personalized blends involves combining carrier oils and essential oils in precise ratios. This allows you to tailor formulations for skincare, massage, or emotional well-being.
- **Holistic wellness**: Together, carrier oils and essential oils contribute to holistic wellness, addressing physical, emotional, and spiritual aspects of well-being. The aromatherapeutic experience combined with the nourishing properties of carrier oils fosters a harmonious connection with nature's botanical treasures.

How to Make Tinctures and Extracts

Tinctures and extracts are potent herbal preparations that harness the medicinal properties of plants for therapeutic use. These liquid formulations are versatile and can be customized to target specific health concerns. We will now explore the art of making tinctures and extracts, outlining the methods, ingredients, and considerations for creating these herbal elixirs.

Choosing Solvents

- Alcohol is commonly used for tinctures due to its excellent extracting properties. High-proof vodka, grain alcohol, or food-grade ethanol is recommended.
- Glycerin is suitable for those avoiding alcohol; it has a sweet taste but may not extract certain compounds as effectively.
- Vinegar is another alcohol-free option suitable for children's preparations, but it may not extract as many constituents as alcohol.

Equipment Needed

- **Glass jars**: Use clean, glass jars with tight-sealing lids for the extraction process. Dark-colored jars help protect the contents from degrading in sunlight.
- **Labels**: Clearly label jars with the ratios of herb(s) and solvent used and the date of preparation.
- **Strainers or cheesecloths**: These are essential for straining the plant material from the liquid after the extraction process. For finely ground herbs, you can use a coffee filter.

Tinctures

Tinctures involve using alcohol as a solvent to extract the active compounds from plant matter. Sometimes, vinegar or glycerin is added to the tincture. Tinctures are highly concentrated and offer a convenient way to administer precise doses without having to consume a lot of liquid. For most tinctures, a common ratio is 1:5 parts herb to alcohol.

How to make a tincture:

1. Grind or cut 3 1/2 oz of fresh or dry herbs into particles measuring roughly 1/8 of an inch, but no more than 3/16 of an inch. This increases the herb's surface area to facilitate better extraction. Do not grind it too finely though, as it will be harder to strain the used herbs out later.
2. Add the herb to a mason jar and cover with 16 fl oz of at least 50-proof alcohol. If the herbs are fresh, use 100-proof alcohol instead as the herbs' water content will dilute the alcohol and therefore the tincture's potency.
3. Seal the jar and shake it vigorously to mix the herbs and solvent well.

4. Store the jar in a cool dark place to macerate. Over 2–4 weeks, shake the jar every day.
5. Strain the tincture to remove all plant parts.

Extracts

An extract is a broad terminology for any substance other than alcohol that has drawn out flavors or active components from a herb. Extracts can be made using solvents like water, glycerin, or vinegar.

How to make an extract:

1. Chop up or grind fresh or dry herbs for maceration—a passive process of extraction.
2. Combine the chopped herbs and menstruum—your chosen solvent—in a glass jar. Ensure the herbs are completely submerged in the menstruum.
3. Store in a cool, dark place, shaking the jar periodically for 2–6 weeks for optimal extraction.
4. After maceration, strain the liquid through a fine mesh strainer or cheesecloth. Squeeze the remaining liquid from the herb material.
5. Pour the strained liquid into dark glass dropper bottles.
6. Label each bottle with the name of the extract, which herbs and solvents were used, and the date.

Crafting Salves, Balms, and Oils

Creating your own herbal oils, salves, and balms allows you to harness the healing properties of plants for skincare, hence, providing nourishment and support to your skin. Calendula, lavender, chamomile, and comfrey are popular choices for skincare.

Equipment Needed

- **Double boiler or heatproof bowl**: for melting and combining ingredients.
- **Stirring utensil**: Wooden or stainless steel spoons work well for mixing.
- **Strainer or cheesecloth**: for straining herbal infusions.
- **Containers**: Choose dark glass jars or tins to protect the products from light.
- **Labels**: Clearly label your containers with the ingredients used and the date of preparation.

Herbal Oils

Creating herbal-infused oils or salves involves extracting active compounds using carrier oils or beeswax. These are often applied topically for skin-related issues.

How to make a cold infusion oil:

1. Finely chop one part herbs and place them in a jar with four parts olive, coconut, jojoba, sunflower, or sweet almond oil.
2. Store the jar in a warm dark place to infuse the oil. Over 2–8 weeks, shake the jar every day.
3. Strain the oil to remove all plant parts.

How to make a warm infusion oil:

1. Finely chop one part herbs and place them in a bowl with four parts olive, sesame, or sunflower oil.
2. Heat the oil to 100°F using a water bath. Keep the temperature at 100°F for 1–5 h. Times may vary depending on the type of herb used.

3. Remove from heat and allow the oil to cool down to room temperature before straining out the plant parts.

Salves and Balms

Salves generally have a soft consistency and absorb into the skin more readily than balms, which makes them perfect for touch-sensitive areas like sunburnt skin and wounds.

Balms have a thicker consistency than salves making them ideal for creating a barrier on the skin like lip balms, and for rubbing into sore muscles.

How to make a salve or balm:

1. Heat your infused oil to 100°F using a water bath. Use four parts infused oil for salves, or one part infused oil for balms.
2. Add one part beeswax to the heated oil and stir the mix until it has melted.
3. Remove from heat and pour into containers while it is still warm.
4. Once the salve or balm has cooled enough to solidify, seal the container.

Capsules and Pills

Herbs can be encapsulated or rolled into pills for convenient oral consumption. This method provides standardized doses.

Equipment Needed

- **Mortar and pestle**: used to grind dried herbs into a fine powder.
- **Empty capsules**: a pair of gelatin halves to fill and compress into capsules.

The Green Glow

- **Capsule maker**: a device for filling multiple capsules simultaneously.
- **Excipient**: the substance that binds herbal pills together.
- **Food dehydrator**: A food dehydrator is optional, although it can significantly speed up the drying process.
- **Containers**: Choose dark glass jars, tins, or other opaque and airtight containers to protect the capsules or pills from light.
- **Labels**: Clearly label your containers with the ingredients used and the date of preparation.

How to make capsules:

1. Powder dry herbs using a mortar and pestle.
2. Fill a capsule maker with empty gelatin capsules. Most capsule makers function in the same way, although some steps may vary.
3. Fill the large side of the capsules with the powdered herb.
4. Use the tamper to tamp down the powder and repeat the second and third step until the capsules are completely filled and compressed.
5. Use the top of the capsule maker to cap the filled bottoms.
6. Store the capsules in an airtight container to prevent humidity from making the capsules sticky. Store away from direct sunlight.

How to make pills:

1. Powder dry herbs using a mortar and pestle. Do not make too much at a time, as the herbs will start losing

their potency as soon as the pills are made. A month's supply is a good amount.

2. Use a 2:1 ratio of herbs to excipient. For the excipient, you can use cocoa butter, coconut oil, glycerin, honey, jaggery, syrup, or water.

3. Slowly add the excipient while kneading the mixture into a thick paste. Ensure the herb and excipient are thoroughly mixed together before proceeding.

4. Roll the mixture into a cylinder 1/2 of an in. thick, and cut it into pieces 1/4 of an in. in size.

5. Shape the pieces into the desired shape and cover them with a dusting of cornstarch to keep them from sticking together.

6. Lay the pills out on parchment paper and allow them to dry in a well-ventilated, dark area; you can also use a food dehydrator.

7. Store pills in an airtight container away from direct sunlight.

Chapter 7

Correct Dosages and Their Importance

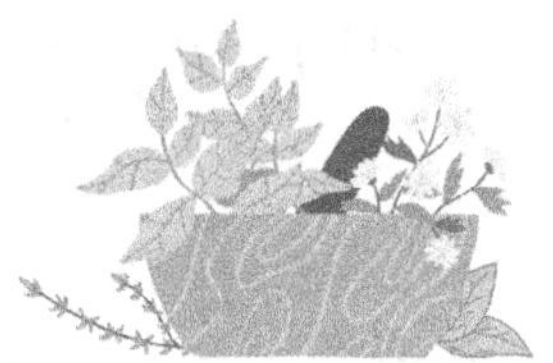

Understanding Potency and Dosage

Knowing the therapeutic properties of herbs is only half of the equation; understanding herbal potency and dosage is the second half and is essential to ensure the safe and effective use of herbal remedies. Next, we will look at the key factors that contribute to herbal potency, methods of preparation, and considerations for determining appropriate dosage.

Factors Influencing Herbal Potency

- **Plant part used**: The roots, leaves, flowers, and seeds may have distinct concentrations of oils and compounds, and therefore varying potency levels. Different parts of a plant contain varying concentrations of active compounds. Some herbal remedies will require the use of a specific part of the plant, as the desired properties may only be present in that part.

- **Growing conditions**: Environmental factors such as soil quality, climate, and altitude can influence the concentration of bioactive compounds in plants.
- **Harvesting time**: The timing of harvesting is crucial to ensure the herb's potency. Some herbs are most potent just before flowering, while others may have peak potency in their leaves, roots, or seeds. Most herbs are best harvested in the morning after the dew evaporates.
- **Storage conditions**: Proper drying and storage of herbs help maintain their potency. Exposure to light, air, and moisture can degrade active compounds.
- **Processing methods**: The way herbs are processed—whether dried, extracted, or prepared in another form—can affect their potency. For example, essential oils extracted through steam distillation are highly concentrated.

Dosage Considerations

Individual Variation

The appropriate dosage can vary from person to person based on factors such as age, weight, overall health, and individual responses to herbs.

Health Conditions

Health conditions may require you to take lower or higher dosages. Herbal remedies can also interact with certain medications. Before taking any herbal medications, you should ask a doctor for medical advice.

Potential allergic reactions to certain herbs must be considered before administering any herbs. For topical use, test a small amount on the skin first and wait a few minutes to see if any reaction occurs.

Purpose of Use

The intended purpose of using herbs influences the dosage. For example, a mild tea for general well-being may have a different dosage than a concentrated tincture for a specific health concern.

Form of Preparation

The potency of different preparations varies. Tinctures and essential oils are more concentrated, therefore, requiring smaller doses than teas or capsules.

Duration of Use

The length of time an individual plans to use an herbal remedy may impact the appropriate dosage. Short-term and long-term use can have different considerations.

Dosage Forms

- **Drops**: Tinctures are often measured in drops. Standardized droppers make it easier to control dosage.
- **Teas and infusions**: Dosage for teas and infusions is typically measured in cups or tablespoons of dried herbs.
- **Capsules and tablets**: Dosage for encapsulated herbs is measured in the number of capsules or tablets taken per day.
- **Topical application**: For oils, salves, or essential oils applied topically, dosage is often measured by the amount applied or the frequency of application.

How Age, Weight, and Overall Health Influence Dosage and Herb Reactions

Considering age, weight, and overall health is integral to the safe and effective use of herbal remedies. These factors play a significant role in determining the appropriate amount of herbs to use, potential reactions, and the overall impact on a person's well-being.

Age

- **Children**: Children often require lower doses of herbs due to their smaller body size and developing physiological systems. Specific herbs may be contraindicated for certain age groups, so it is crucial to consult with a pediatrician or doctor with experience in pediatric herbalism.
- **Adults**: Adults typically have a broader range of dosages, but individual variations still exist. Age-related factors such as metabolic rate and organ function can influence how herbs are processed in the body.
- **Elderly**: Aging can affect metabolism, organ function, and the absorption of nutrients. Elderly individuals may be more sensitive to certain herbs, and caution should be exercised, especially if there are underlying health conditions.

Weight

- **Underweight**: Underweight people may be more sensitive to herbs, as there is less body mass to distribute and metabolize the compounds. Adjusting dosages based on your weight ensures that the concentration of active compounds is appropriate for you.
- **Overweight**: Higher body weight might require larger doses to achieve the desired therapeutic effect. However, individual metabolic factors also play a role,

and it is necessary to consider overall health and metabolism.

Overall Health

Underlying Health Conditions

People with pre-existing health conditions may require tailored herbal approaches and should use herbal remedies with caution. Herbal remedies may exacerbate certain health conditions, so consulting with your doctor is essential.

Organ Function

The organs' health involved in metabolism and excretion such as the liver and kidneys can influence how herbs are processed. Impaired organ function may affect the metabolism and elimination of herbal compounds and lead to them building up in the body.

Individualized Approach

Herbalists often tailor recommendations based on a thorough understanding of the individual's health profile.

Potential Herb Reactions and Safety Considerations

Start Low and Go Slow

It is advisable to start with a low dose and gradually increase it to assess your tolerance and response.

Allergies and Sensitivities

Be aware of potential allergies or sensitivities to specific herbs. Always perform a patch test for topical applications.

Interactions with Medications

Consult with a healthcare professional, especially when using herbs alongside medications, as interactions can occur.

Pregnancy and Nursing

If you are pregnant or nursing, you should exercise caution and consult a doctor before using herbal remedies, as certain herbs may have undesired or potentially dangerous effects for infants. Dosages should be adjusted to ensure safety for both the mother and the developing fetus or breastfeeding infant.

Monitoring Effects

Regularly monitor the effects of herbal remedies. If there are concerns or adverse reactions, discontinue use and seek medical advice.

Digestive Sensitivities

Some herbs may cause digestive discomfort or interact with digestive conditions. Adjusting dosage or choosing alternative herbs may be necessary.

Hormonal Effects

Certain herbs like black cohosh can have hormonal effects, which may be of concern for people with hormonal imbalances or conditions such as PCOS.

Ensuring Safe Consumption and Application

Ensuring the safe consumption and application of herbs involves a combination of research, education, consultation with healthcare professionals, and a personalized approach. Whether ingesting herbal teas, applying herbal preparations topically, or incorporating herbal supplements into your routine, safe consumption and application of herbs are essential for harnessing their therapeutic benefits without adverse effects.

Source High-Quality Herbs

Choose Organic

Whenever possible, opt for organically grown herbs to minimize exposure to pesticides, herbicides, and other contaminants.

Reliable Suppliers

Source herbs from reputable suppliers who adhere to quality standards and provide information on the source, cultivation methods, and potential allergens.

Research and Education

Know Your Herbs

Research each herb thoroughly before use. Understand its properties, potential side effects, interactions with medications, and appropriate dosage.

Stay Informed

Stay updated on the latest research and information about herbal remedies. The field of herbalism is continually evolving, and new findings may influence best practices.

Consultation with Healthcare Professionals

Before Starting New Regimens

Consult with a healthcare professional or herbalist before incorporating new herbs into your routine, especially if you are on medications or have underlying health conditions.

Monitoring

Regularly monitor your health when introducing new herbs. If you experience any unusual symptoms, discontinue use and seek professional advice.

Dosage and Administration

Follow Recommended Dosages

Adhere to recommended dosages provided by healthcare professionals or reputable herbalists or resources. Starting with lower doses allows for individual tolerance assessment.

Tailor Dosages

Adjust dosages based on age, weight, and overall health. Children and the elderly, for instance, may require different doses than adults.

Proper Administration

Pay attention to the form of administration. Topical applications, teas, tinctures, or capsules require different considerations.

Herb Interactions

Multi-Herb Interactions

Consider potential interactions between different herbs when using multiple herbs simultaneously. Some combinations may enhance or counteract each other's effects.

Personalized Approach

Individualized Protocols

Herbal protocols should be individualized based on health goals, preferences, and specific health conditions.

Holistic Considerations

Take a holistic approach by considering lifestyle factors, diet, and overall well-being alongside herbal use.

Storage and Shelf Life

Proper Storage

Store herbs in cool, dark places to preserve their potency. Follow recommended storage guidelines for different forms of herbal preparations.

Check Expiry Dates

Ensure that herbal supplements and preparations have not expired. Using outdated products may result in reduced potency or altered properties. Clearly label all herbal medications with all the relevant information such as the type of herb, date of manufacture, and concentration.

Hygiene and Cleanliness

Clean Preparation Tools

When preparing herbal teas or infusions, ensure that preparation tools are clean to prevent contamination.

Wash Hands

Wash hands thoroughly before handling herbs, especially if working with topical applications.

Wear Gloves

When working with herbs that can be absorbed transdermally (through the skin) it is advisable to wear gloves.

Listen to Your Body

Monitor Reactions

Pay attention to how your body responds to herbal remedies. If you notice any adverse effects, discontinue use and seek professional advice.

Gradual Changes

Introduce new herbs gradually to allow your body to adapt and minimize the risk of unexpected reactions.

Chapter 8

Growing and Harvesting Your Own Herbal Garden

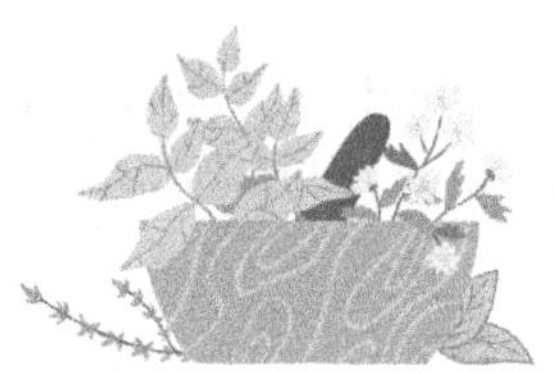

The best way to ensure a regular supply of fresh herbs is to grow your own. Many of the most useful herbs can easily be grown in a home garden. In your very own botanical sanctuary, discover companion planting—a dance of species that repels pests, promotes growth, enhances flavor, and improves the quality of your plants. This chapter will guide you in creating a balanced ecosystem within your herbal sanctuary.

Explore pest control with natural solutions by utilizing companion planting, essential oils, and herbal concoctions to safeguard your garden. Cultivate not only herbs but a harmonious relationship with nature, thus, fostering an environment where health and vitality flourish.

As your garden matures, embrace the art of cultivation—gently coaxing each herb into its fullest expression. Delve into the nuances of soil health, sunlight, and water and become the steward of this green sanctuary. Harvesting becomes a sacred ritual that transforms your efforts into potent elixirs of well-being.

166

30 Easy-to-Grow Plants and How to Grow Them

1. Anise (Pimpinella anisum)

- **growth type**: perennial
- **planting time**: spring after the last frost
- **companion plants**: cilantro, brassicas, legumes, grapes
- **minimum soil temperature to germinate**: 65–70°F
- **sunlight requirements**: full sun
- **planting depth**: 1/4–1/2 in.
- **spacing**: 6–12 in. apart
- **plant size**: 2 ft tall
- **soil type and pH**: well-drained, fertile soil with a pH of 6.3–7.0
- **minimum soil depth**: 12 in.
- **germination time**: 14–21 days
- **feeding schedule**: balanced fertilizer every 4–6 weeks
- **watering**: keep the soil consistently moist
- **time to harvest**: 90–120 days from sowing
- **how to harvest**: harvest the seeds when they turn brown by cutting the seed heads and allowing them to dry

Medicinal Uses

- expectorant
- antispasmodic
- anti-inflammatory
- maintains blood sugar levels
- anti-parasitic

2. Basil (Ocimum basilicum)

- **growth type**: annual
- **planting time**: after the last frost when the soil is warm

- **companion plants**: tomato, pepper, lettuce, carrot, asparagus, cucumber, parsley, cilantro, chives, calendula, lemongrass, marjoram, stinging nettle
- **minimum soil temperature to germinate**: 70°F
- **sunlight requirements**: full sun
- **planting depth**: 1/4 in.
- **spacing**: 12–18 in. apart
- **plant size**: 8 in. tall and wide
- **soil type and pH**: well-drained, fertile, loamy soil with a pH of 6.0–7.5
- **minimum soil depth**: 9–15 in.
- **germination time**: 5–10 days
- **feeding schedule**: balanced fertilizer every 4–6 weeks
- **watering**: keep soil consistently moist
- **time to harvest**: usually 60 days from planting i.e., when the plant has several sets of leaves
- **how to harvest**: harvest individual leaves or cut stems just above a pair of leaves; pinch off growing tips regularly to encourage bushy growth

Medicinal Uses

- headaches
- cough
- diarrhea
- warts
- anti-parasitic

3. Bay (Laurus nobilis)

- **growth type**: perennial
- **planting time**: spring or fall
- **companion plants**: rosemary, lavender, santolina, Mexican daisy

- **minimum soil temperature to germinate**: 70°F
- **sunlight requirements**: full sun to partial shade
- **planting depth**: 1/4 in.
- **spacing**: 12–24 in.
- **plant size**: 1–40 ft tall and wide; wild bay trees can grow up to 60 ft tall
- **soil type and pH**: well-drained, fertile, loamy soil with a pH of 4.5–8.3
- **minimum soil depth**: 12 in.
- **germination time**: 30–90 days
- **feeding schedule**: a balanced fertilizer in spring
- **watering**: water regularly; bay trees prefer consistently moist soil
- **time to harvest**: once the plant is established
- **how to harvest**: as needed; drying is also common for long-term storage

Medicinal Uses

- skin rash
- earache
- rheumatism
- digestive disease
- anti-inflammatory

4. Bee Balm (Monarda didyma)

- **growth type**: perennial
- **planting time**: spring or fall
- **companion plants**: tomato, echinacea, rudbeckia, yarrow, salvia, lavender, catmint, milkweed, comfrey
- **minimum soil temperature to germinate**: 70°F
- **sunlight requirements**: full sun

- **planting depth**: surface sow; seeds need light to germinate
- **spacing**: 18–24 in. apart
- **plant size**: 1–4 ft tall and wide
- **soil type and pH**: well-drained, fertile, loamy soil with a pH of 6.0–7.0
- **minimum soil depth**: 10 in.
- **germination time**: 14–30 days
- **feeding schedule**: early spring with a balanced fertilizer
- **watering**: keep soil consistently moist.
- **time to harvest**: when flowers are in full bloom
- **how to harvest**: cut stems just above a pair of leaves in the morning after the dew has dried but before the heat of the day

Medicinal Uses

- indigestion
- nausea
- UTIs
- menstrual pain relief
- relieves bloating

5. *Borage (Borago officinalis)*

- **growth type**: annual, biennial
- **planting time**: spring
- **companion plants**: tomato, cabbage, squash, strawberry, caraway
- **minimum soil temperature to germinate**: 50–77°F
- **sunlight requirements**: full sun to partial shade
- **planting depth**: 1/4–1/2 in.
- **spacing**: 18–24 in. apart
- **plant size**: 1–3 ft

- **soil type and pH**: well-drained soil with a pH of 4.5–8.5
- **minimum soil depth**: 12 in.
- **germination time**: 7–14 days
- **feeding schedule**: in early spring with a balanced fertilizer
- **watering**: moderate watering, as it is drought-tolerant
- **time to harvest**: 50–60 days from seeding
- **how to harvest**: harvest leaves and flowers as needed; leaves taste best before the plant flowers; flowers are edible and can be used as a garnish or in salads

Medicinal Uses

- anti-inflammatory
- relieves symptoms of asthma
- treats skin conditions such as psoriasis, dermatitis, and eczema
- kidney support
- antidepressant effects

6. Caraway (Carum carvi)

- **growth type**: biennial
- **planting time**: late summer or early spring
- **companion plants**: dill, yarrow, chamomile, borage
- **minimum soil temperature to germinate**: 65°F
- **sunlight requirements**: full sun
- **planting depth**: 1/4–1/2 in.
- **spacing**: 6–12 in. apart
- **plant size**: 8–24 in.
- **soil type and pH**: well-drained, sandy soil with a pH of 6.0–7.5
- **minimum soil depth**: 12 in.

- **germination time**: 14–21 days
- **feeding schedule**: in early spring with a balanced fertilizer
- **watering**: keep soil consistently moist
- **time to harvest**: seeds prepared for harvest in about 90 days
- **how to harvest**: harvest seeds when brown; cut seed heads and dry them

Medicinal Uses

- anti-inflammatory
- aids digestion
- promotes weight loss
- regulates blood sugar
- improves cognitive function

7. Chervil (Anthriscus cerefolium)

- **growth type**: annual, biennial
- **planting time**: early spring or fall
- **companion plants**: lettuce, brassicas, cilantro, dill, yarrow
- **minimum soil temperature to germinate**: 55–65°F
- **sunlight requirements**: partial shade
- **planting depth**: surface sow; seeds need light to germinate
- **spacing**: 6–12 in. apart
- **plant size**: 1–2 ft
- **soil type and pH**: well-drained sandy-loam soil with a pH of 6.5–7.0 and rich in organic matter
- **minimum soil depth**: 12 in.
- **germination time**: 7–14 days

- **feeding schedule**: in early spring with a balanced fertilizer
- **watering**: keep soil consistently moist
- **time to harvest**: at least about 40–60 days after planting
- **how to harvest**: young leaves can be harvested and used fresh; harvest outer leaves first taking care not to damage inner leaves so they can continue growing

Medicinal Uses

- diuretic
- aids digestion
- relieves symptoms of gout
- lowers blood pressure
- anti-inflammatory

8. Chives (Allium schoenoprasum)

- **growth type**: perennial
- **planting time**: spring
- **companion plants**: basil, brassicas, parsley, cilantro, carrots, lettuce, tomatoes, radishes, potatoes, marjoram, rosemary
- **minimum soil temperature to germinate**: 59–68°F
- **sunlight requirements**: full sun to partial shade
- **planting depth**: 1/4 in.
- **spacing**: plant clumps 6–12 in. apart
- **plant size**: 6–18 in. tall
- **soil type and pH**: well-drained soil of pH 6.0–7.0 and rich in organic matter
- **minimum soil depth**: 6–12 in.
- **germination time** 7–14 days
- **feeding schedule**: in early spring with a balanced fertilizer

- **watering**: keep soil consistently moist
- **time to harvest**: leaves can be harvested when the plant is established
- **how to harvest**: snip leaves in clumps with scissors leaving at least 1/2 in. of growth so they can regrow; harvest regularly to encourage new growth

Medicinal Uses

- treats intestinal parasites
- boosts immune systems
- promotes good digestion
- treats anemia
- fights cancer

9. Cilantro (Coriandrum sativum)

- **growth type**: annual
- **planting time**: spring or fall
- **companion plants**: legumes, chervil, brassicas, leafy greens, allium, potato, radish, chives, parsley, basil, lemongrass, stinging nettle
- **minimum soil temperature to germinate**: 65–70°F
- **sunlight requirements**: full sun to partial shade (especially in warmer climates)
- **planting depth**: 1/4 in.
- **spacing**: 6–8 in. apart
- **plant size**: 1–2 ft tall
- **soil type and pH**: well-drained soil of pH 6.5 and rich in organic matter
- **minimum soil depth**: 12 in.
- **germination time**: 7–10 days
- **feeding schedule**: every 4–6 weeks with a balanced fertilizer

- **watering**: keep soil consistently moist
- **time to harvest**: once the plant reaches 6 in. in height
- **how to harvest**: harvest leaves regularly starting from the outer edges and before the plant bolts for the best flavor

Medicinal Uses

- relieves toothache
- reduces the risk of heart disease
- anti-inflammatory
- blood sugar management
- relieves anxiety

10. Comfrey (Symphytum officinale)

- **growth type**: perennial
- **planting time**: spring or fall
- **companion plants**: tomato, mulberry, blueberry, bee balm
- **minimum soil temperature to germinate**: 70°F
- **sunlight requirements**: full sun to partial shade
- **planting depth**: surface sow
- **spacing**: 24–36 in. apart
- **plant size**: 3–4 ft tall and wide
- **soil type and pH**: well-drained soil with a pH of 6.0–7.0; comfrey is adaptable but prefers soil rich in organic matter
- **minimum soil depth**: 18 in.
- **germination time**: 14–21 days
- **feeding schedule**: accumulates nutrients and requires little additional fertilizer
- **watering**: keep the soil consistently moist

- **time to harvest**: leaves can be harvested once the plant is established
- **how to harvest**: cut leaves near the base of the plant, avoiding the flowering stems for better leaf production

Medicinal Uses

- keeps skin healthy
- helps heal sprains, strains, and fractures
- reduces skin inflammation
- treats abrasion wounds
- treats osteoarthritis

11. Dandelion (Taraxacum officinale)

- **growth type**: perennial
- **planting time**: spring or fall
- **companion plants**: broad beans, strawberries, tomatoes, peppers
- **minimum soil temperature to germinate**: 60°F
- **sunlight requirements**: full sun
- **planting depth**: surface sow; do not cover seeds
- **spacing:** 6–12 in. apart
- **plant size**: 18 in.
- **soil type and pH**: well-drained, loamy soil with a pH of around 7.1
- **minimum soil depth**: 8–12 in.
- **germination time**: 7–14 days
- **feeding schedule**: generally not needed for dandelions
- **watering**: keep soil consistently moist. Established plants are drought-tolerant
- **time to harvest**: leaves can be harvested once the plant is established

- **how to harvest**: harvest leaves when young for salads; pick flower heads as soon as they bloom; harvest roots in the fall.

Medicinal Uses

- anti-inflammatory
- regulates blood sugar levels
- reduces cholesterol
- liver support
- lowers blood pressure

12. Dill (Anethum graveolens)

- **growth type**: annual
- **planting time**: late spring or early summer
- **companion plants**: asparagus, brassicas, cucumber, basil, garlic, chervil, valerian
- **minimum soil temperature to germinate**: 60°F
- **sunlight requirements**: full sun
- **planting depth**: 1/4–1/2 in.
- **spacing:** 12–18 in. apart
- **plant size**: 1–4 ft tall
- **soil type and pH**: well-drained soil with a pH of 5.5–6.5
- **minimum soil depth**: 12 in.
- **germination time**: 10–14 days
- **feeding schedule**: balanced fertilizer every 4–6 weeks
- **watering:** only when the top 2 in. of soil is dry
- **time to harvest**: leaves can be harvested once the plant is established, and seeds can be harvested when they turn brown

- **how to harvest**: harvest leaves as needed; collect seeds
  when the flower heads turn brown but before they
  fully open

Medicinal Uses

- reduces the risk of heart disease
- relieves menstrual cramps
- digestive aid
- improves the quality of sleep
- immune system support

13. Echinacea (Echinacea purpurea)

- **growth type**: perennial
- **planting time**: spring or fall
- **companion plants**: bee balm, lavender, yarrow, catmint,
  mulberry, lemongrass
- **minimum soil temperature to germinate**: 70°F
- **sunlight requirements**: full sun to partial shade
- **planting depth**: surface sow; seeds need light to
  germinate
- **spacing**: 18–24 in. apart
- plant size: 2–4 ft tall and 1–2 ft wide
- **soil type and pH**: well-drained, sandy soil with a pH of
  6.0–7.0
- **minimum soil depth**: 12 in.
- **germination time**: 20–30 days
- **feeding schedule**: early spring with a balanced fertilizer
- **watering**: keep the soil consistently moist
- **time to harvest**: roots can be harvested in the fall, and
  flowers can be harvested when fully open
- **how to harvest**: harvest roots in the fall of the second
  year; harvest flowers when fully open for medicinal use

Medicinal Uses

- improves immune function
- relieves pain
- anti-inflammatory
- treats urinary tract infections
- relieves hay fever

14. Fennel (Foeniculum vulgare)

- **growth type**: perennial
- **planting time**: spring or fall
- **companion plants**: lovage, peas, sage
- **minimum soil temperature to germinate**: 60°F
- **sunlight requirements**: full sun
- **planting depth**: 1/4–1/2 in.
- **spacing:** 12–18 in. apart
- **plant size**: 4–6 ft tall and 2–3 ft wide
- **soil type and pH**: well-drained, loamy soil rich in organic matter and with a pH of 6.5–8.0
- **minimum soil depth**: 12 in.
- **germination time**: 7–14 days
- **feeding schedule**: balanced fertilizer every 4–6 weeks
- **watering**: keep soil consistently moist
- **time to harvest**: harvest leaves once the plant is established; seeds can be harvested when they turn brown
- **how to harvest**: harvest leaves as needed; collect seeds when the flower heads turn brown but before they fully open

Medicinal Uses

- relieves digestive discomfort

- eases respiratory issues, including coughs and asthma
- promotes weight loss
- reduces gas and bloating
- promotes milk production for breastfeeding mothers

15. Garlic (Allium sativum)

- **growth type**: perennial
- **planting time**: fall for most regions
- **companion plants**: dill, brassicas, chamomile, yarrow, stinging nettle, tarragon
- **minimum soil temperature to germinate**: 50°F
- **sunlight requirements**: full sun
- **planting depth**: 2 in.
- **spacing:** 4–6 in. apart
- **plant size**: 12–24 in. tall and 2–3 in. wide
- **soil type and pH**: well-drained soil rich in organic matter and with a pH of 5.5–6.5
- **minimum soil depth**: 6 in.
- **germination time**: 7–14 days
- **feeding schedule**: early spring with a balanced fertilizer
- **watering**: keep the soil consistently moist
- **time to harvest**: bulbs are ready when the lower leaves turn brown (usually in late spring or early summer)
- **how to harvest**: dig up bulbs with a garden fork; allow them to cure in a warm, dry place for a few weeks before storing

Medicinal Uses

- supports heart health
- anti-inflammatory
- immune system support
- antibacterial

- detoxifying effects

16. Lavender (Lavandula spp.)

- **growth type**: perennial
- **planting time**: spring or fall
- **companion plants**: echinacea, bee balm, bay, thyme, marjoram, oregano, rosemary
- **minimum soil temperature to germinate**: 70°F
- **sunlight requirements**: full sun
- **planting depth**: surface sow; seeds need light to germinate
- **spacing:** 12–24 in. apart
- **plant size**: 1–3 ft tall and wide
- **soil type and pH**: well-drained, sandy or rocky soil with a pH of 6.5–7.5
- **minimum soil depth**: 12 in.
- **germination time**: 14–21 days
- **feeding schedule**: balanced fertilizer in early spring
- **watering:** only when the top 2 in. of soil is dry; lavender prefers slightly dry conditions
- **time to harvest**: harvest flowers when they are fully open
- **how to harvest**: cut flower spikes just as the buds open for culinary or medicinal use

Medicinal Uses

- promotes relaxation and stress reduction
- improves the quality of sleep
- improves skin health
- relieves headache relief
- relieves anxiety

17. Lemon Verbena (Aloysia citrodora)

- **growth type**: perennial
- **planting time**: spring
- **companion plants**: St. John's wort, lemon balm, cilantro, bee balm, lemongrass, tarragon
- **minimum soil temperature to germinate**: 70°F
- **sunlight requirements**: full sun
- **planting depth**: surface sow
- **spacing:** 12–18 in. apart
- **plant size**: 2–9 ft tall and 3–7 ft wide
- **soil type and pH**: well-drained soil rich in organic matter and with a pH of 6.5
- **minimum soil depth**: 12 in.
- **germination time**: 14–21 days
- **feeding schedule**: balanced fertilizer every 4–6 weeks
- **watering**: keep the soil consistently moist
- **time to harvest**: harvest leaves once the plant is established
- **how to harvest**: snip leaves as needed for culinary or medicinal use

Medicinal Uses

- improves joint function
- anxiety relief and stress reduction
- promotes weight-loss
- anti-inflammatory
- reduces fever

18. Lemongrass (Cymbopogon citratus)

- **growth type**: perennial
- **planting time**: spring or early summer

- **companion plants**: cilantro, basil, thyme, mint, lemon verbena, echinacea
- **minimum soil temperature to germinate**: 70°F
- **sunlight requirements**: full sun to partial shade
- **planting depth**: 1/4–1/2 in.
- **spacing**: 24–36 in. apart
- **plant size**: 2–4 ft tall and wide
- **soil type and pH**: well-drained soil with a pH of 6.0–7.0
- **minimum soil depth**: 8 in.
- **germination time**: 14–21 days
- **feeding schedule**: balanced fertilizer every 4–6 weeks
- **watering**: keep the soil consistently moist
- **time to harvest**: when stalks reach a sufficient size
- **how to harvest**: cut stalks at the base when they are about 1/2 of an in. in diameter for culinary use

Medicinal Uses

- aids digestion
- relieves anxiety
- antiseptic
- relieves pain
- treats skin conditions like dandruff, acne, and eczema

19. Lovage (Levisticum officinale)

- **growth type**: perennial
- **planting time**: spring
- **companion plants**: fennel, hyssop, tomato, beans, catmint
- **minimum soil temperature to germinate**: 60°F
- **sunlight requirements**: full sun
- **planting depth**: surface sow

- **spacing:** 18–24 in. apart
- **plant size:** 4–7 ft tall and 32 in. wide
- **soil type and pH:** moist soil with a pH of 6.5 and rich in organic matter
- **minimum soil depth:** 12 in.
- **germination time:** 14–21 days
- **feeding schedule:** balanced fertilizer every 4–6 weeks
- **watering:** keep the soil consistently moist
- **time to harvest:** harvest leaves and stems once the plant is established
- **how to harvest:** cut leaves and stems as needed for culinary or medicinal use

Medicinal Uses

- kidney support
- aids digestion
- diuretic
- anti-inflammatory
- regulates menstrual cycles

20. Marjoram (Origanum majorana)

- **growth type:** perennial
- **planting time:** spring
- **companion plants:** celery, basil, chives, lavender, parsley, sage, rosemary, thyme, oregano
- **minimum soil temperature to germinate:** 65°F
- **sunlight requirements:** full sun
- **planting depth:** surface sow
- **spacing:** 12–18 in. apart
- **plant size:** 1–2 ft tall
- **soil type and pH:** well-drained soil rich in organic matter and with a pH of 6.9.

- **minimum soil depth**: 6 in.
- **germination time**: 7–14 days
- **feeding schedule**: balanced fertilizer every 4–6 weeks
- **watering**: keep the soil consistently moist. Established plants are drought-tolerant
- **time to harvest**: harvest leaves once the plant is established
- **how to harvest**: cut leaves before the plant flowers; once it has flowered, you can use the flowers

Medicinal Uses

- aids digestion
- improves respiratory health
- promotes relaxation and stress reduction
- anti-inflammatory
- regulates the menstrual cycle

21. Mint (Mentha spp.)

- **growth type**: perennial
- **planting time**: spring or fall
- **companion plants**: tomato, brassicas, carrot, marigold, calendula, chives, garlic, lemongrass
- **minimum soil temperature to germinate**: 72–75°F
- **sunlight requirements**: full sun to partial shade
- **planting depth**: surface sow or cover with a thin layer of soil
- **spacing**: 18–24 in. apart
- **plant size**: 1–4 ft
- **soil type and pH**: moist, well-drained soil
- **minimum soil depth**: 8 in.
- **germination time**: 10–15 days
- **feeding schedule**: usually not necessary

- **watering**: keep the soil consistently moist
- **time to harvest**: harvest leaves once the plant is established
- **how to harvest**: snip leaves as needed for culinary or medicinal use

Medicinal Uses

- relieves Irritable Bowel Syndrome (IBS)
- digestive aid
- improves cognitive function
- promotes weight loss
- reduces the symptoms of asthma

22. Oregano (Origanum vulgare)

- **growth type**: perennial
- **planting time**: spring
- **companion plants**: marjoram, thyme, sage, rosemary, lavender, tarragon
- **minimum soil temperature to germinate**: 72°F
- **sunlight requirements**: full sun
- **planting depth**: surface sow
- **spacing:** 12–18 in. apart
- **plant size**: 1–2 ft tall
- **soil type and pH**: well-drained soil with a pH of 6.5–7.0
- **minimum soil depth**: 8 in.
- **germination time**: 7–14 days
- **feeding schedule**: balanced fertilizer in early spring
- **watering:** only when the top 2 in. of soil is dry
- **time to harvest**: harvest leaves just before flowering
- **how to harvest**: cut stems as needed for culinary or medicinal use

Medicinal Uses

- immune system support
- antibacterial
- anti-inflammatory
- relieves pain
- aids digestion

23. Parsley (Petroselinum crispum)

- **growth type**: biennial
- **planting time**: early spring or late summer
- **companion plants**: apple and pear trees, asparagus, beans, brassicas, marjoram, peppers, tomatoes, tarragon
- **minimum soil temperature to germinate**: 68–80°F
- **sunlight requirements**: full sun to partial shade
- **planting depth**: surface sow
- **spacing:** 6–12 in. apart
- **plant size**: 9–12 in. tall
- **soil type and pH**: well-drained, loamy soil rich in organic matter with a pH of 6.0–7.0
- **minimum soil depth**: 6 in.
- **germination time**: 14–21 days
- **feeding schedule**: balanced fertilizer every 4–6 weeks
- **watering**: keep the soil consistently moist
- **time to harvest**: harvest leaves when the plant is well-established
- **how to harvest**: cut outer leaves as needed for culinary use

Medicinal Uses

- supports kidney health
- fights cancer

- anti-inflammatory
- improves oral health
- aids digestion aid

24. Rosemary (Rosmarinus officinalis)

- **growth type**: perennial
- **planting time**: spring or fall
- **companion plants**: marjoram, oregano, chives, lavender, sage, thyme, strawberry, stinging nettle, tarragon
- **minimum soil temperature to germinate**: 65°F
- **sunlight requirements**: full sun
- **planting depth**: surface sow
- **spacing:** 24–36 in. apart
- **plant size**: 2–6 ft
- **soil type and pH**: well-drained, sandy soil with a pH of 6.0–7.0
- **minimum soil depth**: 10 in.
- **germination time**: 14–21 days
- **feeding schedule**: balanced fertilizer in early spring
- **watering:** only when the top 2 in. of soil is dry
- **time to harvest**: allow rosemary to establish itself in the first year before harvesting; once established, harvest sprigs throughout the growing season
- **how to harvest**: snip sprigs as needed for culinary or medicinal use

Medicinal Uses

- improves cognitive function
- anti-inflammatory
- improves respiratory health
- reduces anxiety

- hair and scalp health

25. Sage (Salvia officinalis)

- **growth type**: perennial
- **planting time**: spring or fall
- **companion plants**: legumes, brassicas, carrot, celery, marjoram, rosemary, oregano, strawberry, tomato, tarragon
- **minimum soil temperature to germinate**: 70°F
- **sunlight requirements**: full sun
- **planting depth**: surface sow
- **spacing:** 18–24 in. apart
- **plant size**: 1–3 ft tall and wide
- **soil type and pH**: well-drained soil with a pH of 6.0–7.0
- **minimum soil depth**: 12 in.
- **germination time**: 14–21 days
- **feeding schedule**: balanced fertilizer in early spring
- **watering**: only when the top 2 in. of soil is dry
- **time to harvest**: harvest leaves once the plant is established
- **how to harvest**: cut leaves before the plant flowers; once it has flowered, you can use the flowers

Medicinal Uses

- improves cognitive function
- soothes sore throat
- reduces symptoms of menopause
- aids digestion
- anti-inflammatory

26. Stinging Nettle (Urtica dioica)

- **growth type**: perennial
- **planting time**: early spring or fall
- **companion plants**: garlic, alfalfa, yarrow, allium, rosemary, cilantro, basil
- **minimum soil temperature to germinate**: 70°F
- **sunlight requirements**: full sun to partial shade
- **planting depth**: surface sow or cover seeds lightly
- **spacing:** 12–18 in. apart
- **plant size**: 3–7 ft
- **soil type and pH**: moist soil with a pH of 6.0–7.0 and rich in organic matter
- **minimum soil depth**: 18 in.
- **germination time**: 7–14 days
- **feeding schedule**: balanced fertilizer in early spring
- **watering**: keep the soil consistently moist
- **time to harvest**: harvest young leaves in spring
- **how to harvest**: wear gloves to avoid stinging, and harvest the top few in. of the plant

Medicinal Uses

- allergy relief
- anti-inflammatory
- diuretic
- improves respiratory health
- increases insulin sensitivity

27. Tarragon (Artemisia dracunculus)

- **growth type**: perennial
- **planting time**: spring or fall

- **companion plants**: Thyme, lemon balm, parsley, rosemary, sage, lemon verbena, garlic, oregano
- **minimum soil temperature to germinate**: 60°F
- **sunlight requirements**: full sun
- **planting depth**: surface sow
- **spacing**: 18–24 in. apart
- **plant size**: 1–3 ft tall
- **soil type and pH**: well-drained soil with a pH of 6.5–7.5
- **minimum soil depth**: 10 in.
- **germination time**: 14–21 days
- **feeding schedule**: balanced fertilizer in early spring
- **watering**: keep the soil consistently moist.
- **time to harvest**: harvest leaves as needed once the plant is established
- **how to harvest**: snip leaves as needed for culinary or medicinal use

Medicinal Uses

- aids digestion
- improves the quality of sleep
- anti-inflammatory
- improves respiratory health
- regulates menstrual cycles

28. Thyme (Thymus vulgaris)

- **growth type**: perennial
- **planting time**: spring or fall
- **companion plants**: potato, tomato, brassicas, rosemary, sage, oregano, marjoram, lavender, lemongrass, tarragon
- **minimum soil temperature to germinate**: 60°F
- **sunlight requirements**: full sun to partial shade

- **planting depth**: surface sow
- **spacing:** 6–12 in. apart
- **plant size:** 6–12 tall and wide
- **soil type and pH**: well-drained, sandy soil with a pH of 6.0–8.0
- **minimum soil depth**: 6 in.
- **germination time**: 7–14 days
- **feeding schedule**: balanced fertilizer in early spring
- **watering:** only when the top 2 in. of soil is dry
- **time to harvest**: harvest stems once the plant is established
- **how to harvest**: cut leaves before the plant flowers; once it has flowered, you can use the flowers

Medicinal Uses

- alleviates respiratory issues, coughs, and congestion
- helps regulate moods
- aids digestion
- anti-bacterial
- immune system support

29. Valerian (Valeriana officinalis)

- **growth type**: perennial
- **planting time**: spring or fall
- **companion plants**: echinacea, catmint, dill, bee balm, chamomile, calendula
- **minimum soil temperature to germinate**: 65–68°F
- **sunlight requirements**: full sun to partial shade
- **planting depth**: surface sow
- **spacing:** 18–24 in. apart
- **plant size:** 2–4 ft tall and wide

- **soil type and pH**: well-drained sandy-loam soil with a pH of 6.0–7.0 and rich in organic matter
- **minimum soil depth**: 18 in.
- **germination time**: 14–21 days
- **feeding schedule**: balanced fertilizer in early spring
- **watering**: keep the soil consistently moist
- **time to harvest**: harvest roots in the fall of the second year
- **how to harvest**: dig up the roots, clean, and dry them for medicinal use

Medicinal Uses

- insomnia
- headaches
- anxiety relief
- relief from symptoms of menopause
- stomach cramps

30. Yarrow (Achillea millefolium)

- **growth type**: perennial
- **planting time**: spring or fall
- **companion plants**: chervil, garlic, echinacea, caraway, bee balm, stinging nettle
- **minimum soil temperature to germinate**: 60°F
- **sunlight requirements**: full sun to partial shade
- **planting depth**: surface sow
- **spacing**: 12–18 in. apart
- **plant size**: 2–3 ft tall
- **soil type and pH**: well-drained, sandy soil with a pH of 5.5–6.8
- **minimum soil depth**: 12 in.
- **germination time**: 14–21 days

- **feeding schedule**: balanced fertilizer in early spring
- **watering:** only when the top 2 in. of soil is dry
- **time to harvest**: harvest flowers and stalks that are in full bloom throughout the growing season
- **how to harvest**: cut flowering stems for culinary or medicinal use

Medicinal Uses

- promotes wound healing
- reduces fever
- relieves menstrual pain
- digestive aid
- anti-inflammatory

Cultivating, Caring for, and Maintaining a Healthy Herbal Garden

Cultivating, caring for, and maintaining a vibrant herbal garden opens the door to a realm where nature's healing wonders flourish right at your fingertips. This endeavor goes beyond the ordinary, inviting you to nurture a sanctuary where your herbal ingredients thrive. We will now delve into the art of growing and sustaining a healthy herbal garden. From soil preparation to strategic care, each step contributes to the vitality of your garden, ensuring a continuous bounty of herbs that not only offer a plethora of medicinal and aromatic delights but also enrich your culinary endeavors.

Selecting a Site for Your Garden

Choose a location with well-drained soil and adequate sunlight for most herbs. Consider the specific sunlight requirements of each herb and plan the garden layout accordingly.

If you have limited garden space, you can successfully grow most herbs on sunny balconies and windowsills using containers.

Soil Testing and Maintaining pH

Before planting or adding soil amendments you should perform a pH test and an electrical conductivity (EC) test on the soil you wish to plant in. These tests are done in order to establish the soil's pH and nutrient levels so that you can calculate the amount of amendments to add. This is best done well in advance to avoid disturbing the roots of established herbs and to allow the amendments to break down and condition the soil before the plants arrive.

Retest the soil once a week until the pH stabilizes before adding more amendments. Avoid adding too much at once as changing soil pH takes some. Continue this process until the desired pH is reached. Slightly acidic to neutral soil with a pH between 6.0 and 7.0 is perfect for most herbs.

Increasing the pH of Acidic Soils

Adding limestone to the soil will slowly raise the pH. Be careful not to overdo it, as it is easier to raise soil pH than to lower it.

Decreasing the pH of Alkaline Soils

Apply elemental sulfur to the soil 3–6 months before planting to allow chemical and biological processes to react with the sulfur to lower the pH.

Soil Amendments

Healthy soil has a good balance of aeration, moisture retention, drainage, and organic matter which promotes a healthy environment for roots and soil microorganisms. Soil amendments are substances added to soil to enhance its fertility, structure, or other physical properties. They play a crucial role in creating an optimal environment for plant growth.

- Improve soil structure by adding organic matter such as compost or well-rotted manure. Organic matter adds nutrients to the soil and improves moisture retention. As organic particles swell and shrink, they break up compacted soil and improve aeration. Apply organic matter regularly or use organic mulches that break down slowly to replenish the soil.
- Mix in perlite or vermiculite to enhance drainage and aeration, especially if the soil is heavy clay.
- Gypsum is a great source of calcium and sulfur that can be added to the soil without changing the pH. It also reduces aluminum toxicity in acidic soils, improves clay soil structure by breaking up compacted soil, improves water infiltration, and reduces the runoff of phosphorus and other nutrients.

Raised Beds

Consider gardening in raised beds, especially if the native soil is poor or drainage is an issue. Raised beds provide better control over soil quality and make gardening more accessible for folks with mobility issues.

Raised bed gardens offer numerous other benefits, such as extending the growing season, offering a natural barrier against some pests, weed reduction, increasing planting density—because of better soil quality—and reducing soil compaction.

Spacing and Arrangement

Space herbs according to their mature size to avoid overcrowding. Plan for easy access and airflow to prevent diseases and simplify maintenance activities, watering, and harvesting.

General Garden Care

Watering

For seedlings and plants that are still establishing themselves, you should water regularly, keeping the soil consistently moist but not waterlogged. Established herbs generally prefer deep, infrequent watering rather than shallow, frequent watering.

The general rule is to water only when the top 2 in. of the soil is dry, but more frequent watering may be necessary for plants in sandy soils or warmer climates.

Mulching

Apply a layer of organic mulch, such as straw or wood chips, to retain moisture and suppress weeds. You can also use landscaping fabric, gravel, or pebbles as mulch.

Mulching also helps regulate soil temperature and provides a barrier against soil-borne diseases.

Fertilizing

Prepare the soil before planting by enriching it with organic matter. For established plants, apply a balanced, organic fertilizer or compost in the spring. Avoid excessive fertilization, as herbs generally prefer lean soil.

Some organic fertilizers worth considering are:

- **Compost and manure**: Compost and animal manure provide essential nutrients and enhance soil structure. Different types of manure, like chicken, cow, or horse manure, offer varying nutrient profiles.
- **Cover crops**: Plants like clover or legumes planted during the off-season help prevent erosion, fix nitrogen, and improve soil structure.

- **Bone meal**: A slow-release phosphorus source derived from animal bones, promoting root development and flowering.
- **Wood ash**: Contains potassium and helps raise soil pH. Use cautiously, as excessive amounts can harm certain plants.
- **Coco coir**: Enhances water retention and aeration, particularly in sandy soils, while adding organic matter.
- **Green manure**: Similar to cover crops, green manure involves planting and incorporating young plants into the soil to improve fertility.
- **Fish emulsion**: A liquid fertilizer made from fish byproducts, rich in nitrogen and other nutrients.
- **Epsom salt**: Supplies magnesium and sulfur, crucial for plant growth, flowering, and fruiting. Epsom salt may even improve the flavor of certain herbs.
- **Vermicompost**: Manure produced by earthworms, providing nutrient-rich organic matter and beneficial microorganisms.

Pruning

Regularly prune or pinch back the tips of herbs to encourage bushier growth and prevent them from becoming leggy.

Promptly prune dead or diseased foliage to curb the spread of pests, fungi, or plant diseases.

Prune excessive growth to improve air circulation, reduce humidity around plants, and prevent fungal diseases.

Weeding

Keep your garden free of weeds that can compete with herbs for nutrients and water. Handpick weeds regularly, especially when they are small, and ensure you remove the roots as well, as some weeds will keep growing back if their roots are left intact.

Maintaining a Healthy Herbal Garden

Disease Prevention

Choose disease-resistant varieties of herbs when possible. Provide adequate spacing and airflow to reduce the risk of fungal diseases.

Regular Inspections

Monitor plants for signs of pests or diseases regularly. Identifying pests, diseases, nutrient deficiencies, and taking prompt action helps prevent issues from spreading.

Support Structures

Install stakes or cages for tall or sprawling herbs to prevent them from falling over. Proper support helps maintain a neat and organized garden while improving airflow and sunlight exposure.

Seasonal Care

Adjust care routines based on the seasons. For example, increase watering during hot summers and reduce it during cooler months. Mulch heavily in winter to protect biennial or perennial herbs from frost.

Propagation

Propagate herbs through cuttings or division to ensure a continuous supply. This practice also helps rejuvenate older plants and maintain overall garden health.

Common Garden Pests

Maintaining a healthy garden can be challenging when faced with various pests that threaten your plants. Early identification of common garden pests is essential for effective pest management. Here is how to recognize and control some of the most prevalent pests that may invade your garden.

Aphids (*Aphidoidea*)

Aphids are small, soft-bodied insects. They are usually green, but can be black, brown, yellow, or pink. Often found in clusters on new growth, buds, or the undersides of leaves, where they extract plant sap, causing leaves to curl, yellow, or distort, weakening plants and transmitting plant viruses. To make matters worse, they excrete a sticky substance called honeydew, promoting the growth of sooty mold.

Control: Use insecticidal soap or neem oil and apply directly to the aphids. Repeat the treatment every other day for two weeks. For a more ecological solution, encourage natural predators like ladybugs or cucumeris (*Neoseiulus cucumeris*), a predatory mite that eats thrips.

Whiteflies (*Aleyrodidae*)

Whiteflies are tiny, moth-like insects with powdery white wings. Like aphids, they can be found on the undersides of leaves in clusters where they feed on plant sap, causing yellowing, wilting, and leaf drop. They excrete honeydew.

Control: Use yellow sticky traps, or introduce natural predators.

Spider Mites (*Tetranychidae*)

Spider mites are extremely small and can sometimes be overlooked. They leave tiny dots in the surface of the leaves they feed on. Webbing may be present between leaves on infested plants. The leaves of heavily infested plants will yellow and die. The mites flourish in hot and dry conditions.

Control: To contain the spread, increase the humidity around plants and use insecticidal soap or neem oil every other day for two weeks. Check nearby plants, as spider mites easily spread around the garden. Introduce natural predators such as cucumeris mites.

Caterpillars (*Lepidoptera larvae*)

Larvae of butterflies or moths have unmistakable segmented bodies with three pairs of legs at the front and more sets of prolegs along its length. They may vary widely in color, size, and appearance, depending on their species. Caterpillars are voracious feeders and chew on leaves, flowers, and stems, quickly defoliating plants.

Control: Handpick caterpillars off of plants and dispose of them. Continue to monitor your plants for any more caterpillars. For biological control, apply *Bacillus thuringiensis* (Bt), a soil-dwelling bacteria toxic to caterpillars but safe for humans and other mammals.

Slugs and Snails (*Gastropoda*)

Snails are soft-bodied, slimy mollusks with shells on their backs, while slugs are similar mollusks with an internalized soft shell. They are most active at night and on cloudy or rainy days when they come out of hiding to eat irregular holes in leaves and stems. Slime trails on plants and soil are telltale signs of snail and slug activity.

Control: Handpick these mollusks or use beer traps to lure them. Applying diatomaceous earth or copper barriers around plants prevents snails and slugs from crossing.

Japanese Beetles (*Popillia japonica*)

These beetles are metallic green and bronze with distinctive white tufts along their side. They feed in groups, skeletonizing leaves and damaging flowers and fruit. They attract more beetles to the feeding site through pheromones.

Control: Handpick or brush the beetles into soapy water. Place Japanese beetle traps some distance away from your plants to lure the insects away.

Cutworms (*Noctuidae larvae*)

Cutworms are smooth, plump caterpillars, often found curled up under fallen debris when at rest. They are most active at night when they cut through plant stems at ground level. Young seedlings are particularly vulnerable to cutworms.

Control: Prevent cutworms from getting to your plants by clearing the bases of your plants of fallen debris and leaf litter and using collars around seedlings. Apply a biological pesticide.

Thrips (*Thysanoptera*)

Thrips are small, slender insects, often yellow, brown, or black. They feed in groups, sucking plant sap and leaving behind a stippled appearance on leaves. The leaves of heavily infested plants will become pale or mottled with distorted growth. Like other sap-sucking pests, thrips can transmit diseases between plants.

Control: Use insecticidal soap or neem oil and spray directly on the pests. Introduce natural predators like predatory mites.

Scale Insects (*Coccoidea*)

These are small, immobile insects with a protective shell. Different species of scale insects come in a variety of colors, shapes, and textures. They usually remain in one spot on the stems and undersides of leaves where they drain plant sap, causing yellowing, wilting, and leaf drop. Like aphids, they produce honeydew that leads to sooty mold.

Control: Use insecticidal soap, neem oil, or introduce natural predators.

Fungus Gnats (*Sciaridae*)

Fungus gnats are small, mosquito-like insects with long legs. Although the adult gnats do not harm plants, their larvae feed on plant roots, causing distorted growth and death.

Control: Use insecticidal soap or neem oil and spray directly on the gnats. Use yellow sticky traps, or introduce natural predators like Sciarid fly nematodes.

Pest Prevention and Control Methods

Managing the various pests that can threaten plants is key to maintaining a healthy garden. A combination of pest control methods preventive measures, biological controls, and, in some cases, chemical interventions tailored to the specific needs and conditions of your garden, can create a balanced and effective approach to pest management. Integrated Pest Management (IPM) encourages a holistic strategy that minimizes environmental impact while maintaining a healthy garden ecosystem. Always consider the potential risks and benefits of each method, aiming for the least harmful interventions whenever possible.

Preventive Measures

- **Crop rotation**: Rotating crops each season helps disrupt the life cycle of pests that target specific plant species.
- **Proper watering and fertilization**: Maintaining optimal watering and fertilization practices helps keep plants healthy and more resistant to pests.
- **Healthy soil**: Well-balanced soil with proper organic matter supports robust plant growth and can deter certain pests.

- **Mulching**: Mulching around plants helps retain moisture, suppress weeds, and create a barrier that can deter some pests.
- **Proper spacing:** Planting at recommended distances helps reduce the risk of diseases spreading and makes it harder for pests to move between plants.
- **Proper watering:** Water in the morning to allow foliage to dry during the day and water plants at the base rather than overhead to minimize conditions favorable for fungal diseases and pests.
- **Adequate nutrition**: Maintain balanced soil fertility to ensure plants are healthy and less susceptible to pest infestations.
- **Remove infected plants**: Promptly remove and dispose of plants that show signs of disease or severe pest damage. Do not compost any of this material to prevent contaminating your garden again.
- **Provide habitat for predators**: Maintain areas with native plants and shelter to encourage natural predators like ladybugs, spiders, and predatory wasps. Herbs like dill are a favorite habitat for predatory insects.
- **Clean garden tools**: Regularly clean and disinfect gardening tools to prevent the spread of diseases. When pruning diseased foliage, do not cut any other plants until you have disinfected the cutting implements.
- **Remove garden debris**: Eliminate hiding places for pests by regularly removing fallen leaves, weeds, and other debris.
- **Regular monitoring**: Regularly inspect plants for signs of pests or diseases. Early detection allows for prompt intervention.
- **Research local pests and diseases**: Stay informed about local pests and diseases, enabling you to anticipate potential issues and take preventive measures.

Biological Control

- **Beneficial insects**: Introduce predatory insects like ladybugs and lacewings that feed on pests.
- **Nematodes**: Use beneficial nematodes to control soil-dwelling pests like grubs and larvae.
- **Predatory mites**: Deploy predatory mites to control spider mite populations.
- **Parasitoids**: Release parasitoid wasps that lay eggs on or inside pests, eventually killing them.
- **Birds and bats**: Encourage birds and bats in the garden, as they feed on various pests.

Mechanical and Physical Controls

- **Handpicking**: Physically removing pests by hand is effective for larger insects like caterpillars or beetles.
- **Traps**: Yellow sticky traps attract and capture flying insects like whiteflies, aphids, thrips, and fungus gnats.
- **Row covers**: Use floating row covers to physically protect plants from flying pests and reduce the risk of infestations.
- **Netting**: Install netting to protect crops from birds, rabbits, and larger pests.
- **Pruning**: Prune and remove infested plant parts to control the spread of pests and diseases.
- **Water spray**: Spraying plants with a strong stream of water can dislodge and remove pests like aphids and spider mites, however, this is only a temporary solution.

Cultural Controls

- **Timing of planting**: Planting a little later in spring can help avoid peak pest seasons.

- **Resistant varieties**: Choose plant varieties that are naturally resistant to common pests in your area.
- **Diversify plantings**: Mix different plant species to create a diverse ecosystem, making it more challenging for pests to establish.
- **Trap crops**: Planting specific crops to attract pests away from the main crops can help protect the primary plants.
- **Companion planting**: Plant crops together that help deter pests or attract beneficial insects that prey on pests. Plant aromatic herbs like basil and mint to repel certain pests.

Chemical Controls

- **Insecticidal soaps**: Soaps disrupt the cell membranes of insects, controlling pests like aphids, whiteflies, and spider mites.
- **Neem oil**: Neem oil acts as a natural insecticide and fungicide, controlling a broad spectrum of pests.
- **Botanical pesticides**: Derived from plants, substances like pyrethrin (from chrysanthemums) can be effective against certain pests.
- **Chemical insecticides**: Synthetic chemical pesticides should be used as a last resort due to potential environmental impact and harm to beneficial insects.
- **Systemic pesticides**: Applied to the soil or foliage, systemic pesticides are absorbed by plants and can control pests that feed on them.

Integrated Pest Management (IPM)

- **Monitoring**: Regularly inspect plants for signs of pests and their damage.

- **Thresholds**: Determine acceptable pest levels and take action if thresholds are exceeded.
- **Record keeping**: Maintain records of pest populations, interventions, and outcomes for future planning.
- **Sustainable practices**: Emphasize ecological and sustainable pest management strategies.
- **Regular evaluation**: Continuously evaluate and adjust pest control strategies based on their effectiveness.

Homemade Sprays

Create homemade sprays using ingredients like neem oil, castile soap, garlic, onion, tobacco, or cayenne pepper infusions to deter or eliminate pests.

- **Garlic spray**: Crush a garlic bulb or add two tablespoons of garlic powder, and one tablespoon of castile soap to 40 ounces of water and leave to soak for 24 hours.
- **Onion spray**: Boil the outer layers and skins from three onions in half a gallon of water for 5–10 minutes, then add another half a gallon of water and allow the skins to soak in the water for a week before straining them out.
- **Tobacco spray**: Soak one cup of dried tobacco in a gallon of water overnight and strain the tobacco out.
- **Bicarbonate of soda spray**: Controls and helps eliminate pests like aphids, thrips, and spider mites, and to prevent and manage fungal diseases like powdery mildew. To make this spray, simply mix one tablespoon of bicarbonate of soda with one gallon of water and add one teaspoon of castile soap. Do not overuse bicarbonate of soda, as it can lead to high salt levels in the soil.

The Harvest: When and How to Gather Herbs

Harvesting herbs is both an art and a science. When you harvest herbs at the right time and use the proper techniques you ensure that the herbs have the maximum flavor, aroma, and medicinal properties you require. By understanding the growth habits of different herbs, recognizing optimal harvest times, and employing proper techniques, you can enjoy a bountiful harvest of flavorful, aromatic, and healthful herbs. Always approach harvesting with care and consideration for the plants' well-being to ensure a continuous supply throughout the growing season. Adhering to the following guide on when and how to gather herbs will ensure that you get the best results.

Timing the Harvest

- **Early morning**: Harvest herbs early in the morning just after the dew has evaporated. This is the time of day when essential oils are at their peak concentration. Harvesting later in the day may cause your herbs to wilt in the midday sun.
- **Before flowering**: Harvest herbs before they flower as this is when their flavors are most intense. Once herbs start flowering, the energy may shift from leaves to seeds, altering taste. Some leafy herbs like basil and parsley become bitter after flowering.
- **Perennial herbs**: For perennial herbs, harvest sparingly in the first year, allowing the plants to establish. In subsequent years, harvests can be more generous.

Tools for Harvesting

- **Clean and sharp scissors or pruners**: Use clean and sharp scissors or pruners to make precise cuts without damaging the plant.

- **Harvesting basket**: Carry a harvesting basket to collect herbs, allowing for proper air circulation and preventing bruising.
- **Gloves**: Wear gloves if harvesting herbs with sap or oils that may cause skin irritation.
- **Clean cloth, paper towel, or soft brush**: Clean any dirt or debris from the harvested herbs gently using a clean cloth, paper towel, or brush. Do not wash or rinse herbs

Harvesting Techniques

- **Pinching**: Pinch or snip the tips of herb stems for bushier growth. Leaves will branch out where the growing tips have been removed. This is particularly effective for basil, mint, and oregano.
- **Cut above leaf nodes**: Use clean scissors or pruners to cut above leaf nodes of tougher stems to encourage branching and fuller plants.
- **Leave some growth**: Harvest regularly but avoid stripping the plant entirely. Harvest no more than one-third of the plant at once to ensure the plant has enough foliage to bounce back and ensure healthy growth and continued harvests.

Harvesting Specific Types of Herbs

- **Leafy herbs**: Harvest the leaves of leafy herbs like basil, mint, and cilantro before flowering for the best flavor. Regular harvesting also prevents plants from becoming woody.
- **Woody herbs**: Harvest woody herbs like rosemary, thyme, and lavender) in the morning after the dew has

evaporated. Trim the tips of branches to promote denser growth.

- **Root herbs**: Harvest root herbs like ginger, and turmeric when the leaves begin to yellow and die back. Dig carefully around the base with a garden fork or trowel to avoid damaging the roots.
- **Seed-producing herbs**: Harvest seeds from herbs like dill, fennel, and cilantro (coriander) when they are fully mature but before they drop. Cut seed heads and allow them to dry in a well-ventilated area before collecting seeds.
- **Flowering herbs**: Harvest flowering herbs like echinacea, chamomile, and lavender as they start to bloom or during flowering when concentrations of active compounds are at their highest.

Drying and Storing Herbs

- **Air drying**: Tie small bunches of herbs together and hang them upside down in a well-ventilated, dry area. Avoid direct sunlight to preserve color and essential oils.
- **Dehydrator**: Use a dehydrator for faster and more controlled drying of herbs.
- **Storage containers**: Store dried herbs in airtight containers away from heat and light to maintain freshness.
- **Refrigeration**: Store fresh herbs in the fridge for up to 3 weeks
- **Freeze for longevity**: Freeze herbs in ice cube trays with water or olive oil for an even longer shelf life—up to 12 months! Note that olive oil only starts to freeze solid at 10°F.

Chapter 9

Recipes for the New Herbal Enthusiast

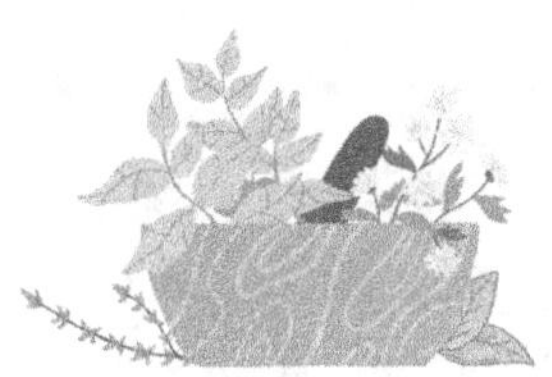

The Benefits of Cooking With Herbs and Spices

Long before you picked up this book, you have been enjoying the benefits of herbs and spices. Not only did they improve your dishes by adding flavor and aroma but they have also been quietly healing you! The benefits of cooking with herbs and spices are many and diverse.

Medicinal Properties

Many herbs and spices possess medicinal properties and have been traditionally used for their health benefits. Incorporating them into your cooking allows you to enjoy their therapeutic effects while savoring delicious meals. For example, turmeric is renowned for its anti-inflammatory properties, and garlic is known for its immune-boosting qualities.

Nutrient Boost

Herbs and spices contain a lot of minerals, vitamins, and antioxidants. Adding them to your recipes not only imparts flavor but also contributes essential nutrients to your diet. For instance, parsley is high in vitamin K and C, while cinnamon is a potent source of antioxidants.

Digestive Support

Certain herbs and spices aid in digestion. Ingredients like ginger and peppermint can help alleviate digestive discomfort, reduce bloating, and promote overall digestive well-being.

Blood Sugar Regulation

Some herbs and spices such as cinnamon and fenugreek have been linked to helping regulate blood sugar levels. This can be particularly beneficial for individuals managing conditions like diabetes.

Anti-Microbial Properties

Many herbs and spices exhibit innate anti-microbial properties that combat bacteria and other microorganisms including garlic, thyme, and oregano.

Heart Health

Certain herbs including rosemary and basil have been associated with heart-protective benefits. They may help in managing cholesterol levels and supporting cardiovascular health.

Weight Management

Herbs and spices can add flavor to dishes without the need for excessive salt, sugar, or unhealthy fats. This can be advantageous for those aiming to manage their weight or make nutritious food more appealing.

Mood Enhancement

The aroma and flavor of herbs and spices can have a positive impact on mood. For instance, the scent of lavender or the taste of saffron may contribute to feelings of relaxation and well-being.

Culinary Creativity

Cooking with herbs and spices allows for endless culinary creativity. Herbalists appreciate the diverse range of flavors, textures, and aromas these botanicals bring to dishes, making meals not only nourishing but also a sensory delight.

Recipes Using Multiple Herbs

Herb Salad (Four Servings)

Ingredients

- 2 cups dandelion greens
- 3 cups watercress leaves
- ½ cup parsley
- ¼ cup chives
- ¼ cup chervil
- 4 minced medium garlic cloves
- ¼ teaspoon sea salt
- ½ teaspoon ground black pepper
- 2 teaspoon Dijon-style mustard
- 3 tablespoons olive oil
- 1 tablespoon red wine vinegar

Utensils

- medium bowl
- small bowl

The Green Glow

Instructions to Make the Salad

1. Chop all the greens into bite-sized pieces.
2. Mix them all together.

Instructions to Make the Vinaigrette

1. In a separate bowl, add the minced garlic to the other ingredients and whisk them together until they are mixed well.
2. Dress the salad with the vinaigrette and serve.

Dandelion Scones (Eight Servings)

Ingredients

- 2 cups all-purpose flour
- 1 tablespoon baking powder
- 1/2 teaspoon sea salt
- 1/3 cup golden honey
- 5 tablespoons chilled unsalted butter
- 1 cup heavy cream
- 1 cup dandelion petals
- 1 cup minced lemon balm

Utensils

- large bowl
- round 9 in. cake pan

Instructions

1. Preheat the oven to 450°F and position the rack in the middle.

2. In a large bowl, mix together the baking powder, sea salt, and flour.
3. Fold the honey into the dry mix.
4. Add the butter to the mix until it has a coarse cornmeal texture.
5. Add the dandelion petals and lemon balm.
6. Mix the heavy cream in until it forms a dough.
7. Transfer the dough to a floured surface and knead for 5–10 s.
8. Press the dough into the cake pan.
9. Flip the pan upside down to remove the shaped dough.
10. Cut the dough into 8 equal wedges.
11. Place the wedges on a cookie sheet and bake for 12–15 min while rotating the pan halfway through until the tops of the scones turn golden brown.
12. Let the scones rest and cool for 10 min before serving.

Elderberry Syrup for Immune Health (Three Servings)

Ingredients

- 2 cups of elderberries
- 4 cups of water
- 2–3 teaspoons ginger root
- 1 cinnamon stick
- 1 cup raw honey

Utensils

- medium pot
- strainer or cheesecloth

Instructions

1. Add the berries, herbs, and cold water to a pot and bring it to a boil.
2. Lower the heat and let it simmer for 30–40 min.
3. Remove from heat and allow it to steep for an hour.
4. Strain out the herbs, squeezing them to get all the juices out.
5. Add the honey and stir the mixture well.

Coconut Vanilla Cardamom Granola (15 Servings)

Ingredients

- 2 cups whole oats
- 1 cup coconut flakes
- 1 cup pumpkin seeds
- 1/2 cup whole almonds
- 1/3 cup hemp seeds
- 1 1/2 teaspoon cardamom powder
- 1 teaspoon cacao powder
- 1 pinch of ground black pepper
- 1/3 cup raw honey
- 1/4 cup coconut oil
- 2 tablespoons Maple syrup
- 1/2 teaspoon vanilla extract

Utensils

- large bowl
- smaller bowl
- oven pan

Instructions

1. Preheat the oven to 275°F.
2. Mix the dry ingredients together in the large bowl.
3. Mix the wet ingredients in a separate bowl.
4. Pour the wet mix over the dry mix and stir together until everything is evenly coated.
5. Spread the mixture out into an oven pan and bake.
6. Stir the contents of the pan every 10 min for 45 min or until the coconut flakes turn golden brown.
7. Allow the granola to cool before storing it in an airtight container.

Paleo Ashwagandha Chocolate Chai Bites (16 Bites)

Ingredients

- 1/3 cup tahini
- 1/4 cup + 1 tablespoon nut butter
- 1/4 cup + 2 tablespoons raw honey
- 1/4 cup chopped dark chocolate
- 2 tablespoons ashwagandha powder
- 2 tablespoons cacao powder
- 2 tablespoons hemp seeds
- 1 teaspoon cinnamon powder
- 1 teaspoon ginger powder
- 1 teaspoon cardamom powder
- 1 teaspoon nutmeg powder
- 1/2 teaspoon vanilla extract

Utensils

- large bowl

Instructions

1. Mix the tahini, nut butter, and honey in a large bowl until it is smooth.
2. Add the herb powders and mix.
3. Add the vanilla extract, hemp seeds, and chocolate.
4. Add more cacao until the dough is thick and does not stick to the sides of the bowl.
5. Break pieces off the dough ball and roll into 1-inch balls.
6. Coat the balls with coconut flakes or hemp seeds.

Caraway Sauerkraut (Eight Servings)

Ingredients

- 1 lbs cabbage
- 2 teaspoons fine sea salt
- 1 tablespoon caraway seeds

Utensils

- fermentation jar
- fermentation seal
- glass weights
- large bowl

Instructions

1. Cut the cabbage in half, remove its core, and slice the cabbage into 1/8 in. thick strips.
2. Mix the cabbage, sea salt, and caraway seeds together in a large bowl.

3. Let it stand for 20 min so the cabbage can soften up. If necessary, squeeze the cabbage to release more juice.
4. Fill a fermentation jar with sauerkraut, and pack it tightly so no bubbles remain and the cabbage is completely submerged in its juice.
5. Weigh the sauerkraut down with a glass fermentation weight to ensure the cabbage remains submerged.
6. Seal the jar and store it for a month at room temperature and away from direct sunlight.

Einkorn Gingerbread (16 servings)

Ingredients

- 2 cups all-purpose einkorn flour
- 1/4 cup unrefined sugar
- 1 teaspoon baking soda
- 1/2 teaspoon fine sea salt
- 1 teaspoon ground cinnamon
- 1/4 teaspoon powdered cloves
- 1/4 teaspoon ground cardamom
- 1/2 cup melted salted butter
- 2 tablespoons grated ginger
- 3/4 cup light molasses
- 1 beaten egg
- 1 cup buttermilk
- 1/4 cup diced, candied ginger

Utensils

- square 9 in. baking pan
- large bowl
- medium bowl
- whisk or electric mixer

The Green Glow

Instructions

1. Preheat the oven to 350°F.
2. Grease the baking pan.
3. Whisk the flour, sugar, salt, baking soda, cloves, cardamom, and cinnamon together.
4. In a different bowl, whisk the molasses, buttermilk, ginger, and melted butter together.
5. Mix the wet and dry ingredients and beat until it forms a smooth batter.
6. Fold in the candied ginger.
7. Pour the batter into the baking pan.
8. Bake for 30–35 min.
9. Allow it cool in the pan for 5 min before removing it from the pan. Allow to cool completely.
10. Dust the cake lightly with some powdered sugar, cut it into 16 equal pieces, and serve.

Simple Tea Blends, Salves, and Balms

Simple Tea Blends

An herbal tea blend can include multiple herbs and is usually formulated using three parts of a base element, two parts of a support element, and one part accent element. Feel free to adjust the ratios based on your taste preferences and experiment with the following blends to create your own unique herbal infusions:

Calm and Relax Blend

- chamomile
- lemon balm
- lavender

Digestive Aid Blend

- peppermint
- ginger
- fennel

Energizing Citrus Blend

- lemongrass
- orange peel
- spearmint

Immune Booster Blend

- echinacea
- elderberry
- rosehip

Sleepy Time Blend

- valerian root
- passionflower
- skullcap

Detoxifying Blend

- dandelion root
- burdock root
- nettle

Spiced Chai Blend

- cinnamon

The Green Glow

- cardamom
- cloves

Minty Fresh Breath Blend

- peppermint
- spearmint
- parsley

Focus and Clarity Blend

- gotu kola
- ginkgo biloba
- rosemary

Salves and Balms

Using the methods discussed in Chapter 6, you can craft these salves and balms:

Salve for Mild Burns and Scrapes

1. Use equal parts comfrey leaf, oregon grape root, and calendula to create a herb-infused oil.
2. Gently heat four parts of infused oil and melt one part beeswax into it.
3. Add a drop of lavender essential oil per 4 fl oz of infused oil.
4. Pour into a container to allow it to set.

Salve for Rashes

1. Use equal parts lemon balm, chamomile, and marshmallow root to create a herb-infused oil.

2. Gently heat four parts of infused oil and melt one part beeswax into it.
3. Add a drop of sage essential oil per 4 fl oz of infused oil.
4. Pour into a container to allow it to set.

Chapter 10

Expanding Your Herbal Horizons

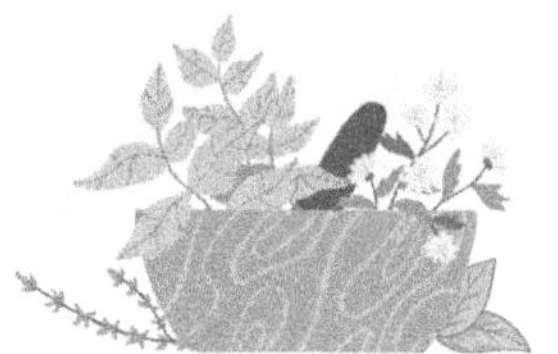

Recommended Literature and Influential Herbalists

With deep roots in nearly every culture around the world, herbalism has a wealth of knowledge that has been passed down through countless generations. Many influential herbalists have contributed to the field passing on their wealth of knowledge to the world. In modern times, a plethora of books have been written on the subject with each new generation contributing more knowledge and valuable insights to demystify the field of herbalism.

Modern Literature on Herbalism

- ***The Complete Illustrated Holistic Herbal* by David Hoffmann**: A comprehensive guide that covers the principles and practices of herbal medicine including herbal actions, energetics, and therapeutic uses.
- ***The Herbal Medicine-Maker's Handbook* by James Green**: An excellent resource for those interested in

preparing their herbal remedies covering the basics of making tinctures, salves, and other herbal preparations.

- ***The Modern Herbal Dispensatory* by Thomas Easley and Steven Horne**: This book provides a modern approach to herbal medicine blending traditional wisdom with contemporary herbal practices.

- ***Herbal Medicine From the Heart of the Earth* by Sharol Tilgner**: Dr. Tilgner's book explores herbal medicine from a clinical perspective offering practical insights into diagnosis and herbal treatment.

- ***The Complete Medicinal Herbal: A Practical Guide to the Healing Properties of Herbs* by Penelope Ody**: This tome delves into the history of herbalism describing ancient uses and properties of herbs, and includes stunning images and detailed how-to methods for creating herbal remedies.

- ***The Herbalist's Way: The Art and Practice of Healing with Plant Medicines* by Nancy and Michael Phillips**: A guide that not only provides herbal knowledge but also emphasizes the spiritual and intuitive aspects of herbalism.

- ***Botany in a Day: The Patterns Method of Plant Identification* by Thomas J. Elpel**: An essential resource for herbalists interested in plant identification, this book teaches a systematic approach to recognizing plant families.

- ***The Essential Margaret Roberts: My 100 Favourite Herbs* by Margaret Roberts**: Drawing from a lifetime of cultivating herbs and practicing herbal medicine, Roberts details how to design a herbal garden, how to cultivate 100 of her favorite herbs, as well as how to craft with herbs.

Influential Herbalists of the 20th and 21st Century

- **Rosemary Gladstar**: Renowned herbalist, teacher, and author of many books on herbs, Rosemary Gladstar has played a pivotal role in popularizing herbalism in the United States. She founded the California School of Herbal Studies and the United Plant Savers.
- **Matthew Wood**: A practicing herbalist and author, Wood is known for blending traditional Western herbalism with a constitutional approach, focusing on the person's unique characteristics.
- **Susun Weed**: An herbalist, author, and teacher, Susun Weed emphasizes the Wise Woman Tradition, which celebrates the healing power of local plants and simple remedies.
- **Michael Tierra**: A prominent herbalist and acupuncturist, Tierra founded the American Herbalists Guild. His contributions include books like *The Way of Herbs* and *The Herbal Tongue*.
- **Matthew Becker**: An ethnobotanist and herbalist, Becker has worked with indigenous cultures to preserve traditional herbal knowledge. His book Rural Plant Medicine explores the traditional uses of plants in rural communities.
- **David Winston**: A clinical herbalist and ethnobotanist, Winston has been influential in integrating traditional herbalism with scientific research. He co-authored *Adaptogens: Herbs for Strength, Stamina, and Stress Relief*.
- **Aviva Romm**: A physician, herbalist, and midwife, Dr. Romm combines conventional medicine with herbalism. Her book *Botanical Medicine for Women's Health* is a valuable resource in women's herbal health.

Traditional Texts

- ***The Complete Herbal* by Nicholas Culpeper**: An influential work from the 17th century, Culpeper's herbal tome provides a historical perspective on herbal medicine.
- ***Hippocratic Corpus***: A collection of ancient Greek medical texts attributed to Hippocrates, this work includes writings on herbal medicine and the principles of healing.
- ***Shennong Ben Cao Jing (Shennong's Materia Medica)***: An ancient Chinese textattributed to Shennong—an ancient Chinese deity—it catalogs numerous medicinal plants.
- ***Dioscorides' De Materia Medica***: A work by Dioscorides—a Greek physician, pharmacologist, and botanist—that served as a significant herbal reference in the ancient world.

The world of herbalism is vast and continually evolving. Exploring historic and modern literature on herbs and learning from influential herbalists can provide a solid foundation in traditional and modern herbal practices. These resources offer a blend of practical knowledge, scientific understanding, and cultural perspectives, making them valuable for both beginners and seasoned herbalists seeking to deepen their understanding of plant medicine.

Emphasizing Cross-Cultural Respect in Global Herbal Practices

Herbal practices are deeply rooted in diverse cultural traditions worldwide each with its unique perspectives, knowledge, and approaches to healing. Emphasizing cross-cultural respect in global herbal practices, acknowledging the richness of various traditions, and ensuring that herbalism is practiced ethically and inclusively is essential for collaboration and effectiveness.

Importance of Cross-Cultural Respect

Through cross-cultural respect, herbal practices can thrive as a collective tapestry of global healing traditions.

Preservation of Traditional Knowledge

Many herbal traditions are transmitted orally and through generations. Cross-cultural respect ensures the preservation of traditional knowledge, thus, preventing its loss due to appropriation or exploitation.

Cultural Sensitivity

Recognizing and respecting diverse cultural practices demonstrates cultural sensitivity. It acknowledges that herbalism is deeply intertwined with cultural identity and heritage.

Avoiding Cultural Appropriation

Cross-cultural respect encourages herbal practitioners to be mindful of the potential for cultural appropriation. It prompts a thoughtful approach, ensuring that practices are not taken out of context or used without understanding their cultural significance.

Holistic and Inclusive Healthcare

Embracing diverse herbal traditions contributes to the development of a more holistic and inclusive approach to healthcare. Different cultures offer unique insights into the relationships between plants, individuals, and communities.

Promoting Global Collaboration

Cross-cultural respect reinforces global collaboration among herbalists, researchers, and practitioners. This collaboration can lead to the exchange of new knowledge, innovative practices, and mutual learning.

Respecting Sacred and Ritual Practices

Many herbal traditions include sacred or ritualistic elements. Cross-cultural respect acknowledges and respects these practices, thereby understanding their significance beyond medicinal use.

Enhancing Herbal Diversity

Different regions have unique ecosystems that support diverse plant life. Cross-cultural respect encourages the exploration and appreciation of herbal diversity, therefore, recognizing the value of various plants across cultures.

Ways to Promote Cross-Cultural Respect in Herbal Practices

Learn from Diverse Sources

Expand your herbal knowledge by learning from diverse sources including texts, practitioners, and communities from different cultural backgrounds.

Cultural Competency Training

Herbal practitioners can undergo cultural competency training to better understand and respect the cultural contexts of the herbal traditions they engage with.

Engage in Intercultural Exchanges

Attend conferences, workshops, or events that bring together herbalists from various cultural backgrounds. Engaging in intercultural exchanges promotes understanding and collaboration.

Consult and Collaborate

When working with herbs from a culture different than your own, consult with or collaborate with practitioners from that culture. Seek their guidance to ensure respectful and accurate use of herbal knowledge.

Acknowledge Cultural Intellectual Property

Respect intellectual property rights and acknowledge the cultural ownership of herbal knowledge. Give credit to the originators of specific practices or remedies.

Use Inclusive Language

When discussing herbal practices, use inclusive language that acknowledges the diversity of cultural perspectives. Avoid generalizations that may oversimplify or misrepresent cultural practices.

Support Indigenous Rights

Advocate for the rights of indigenous communities to control and benefit from the use of traditional herbal knowledge. Respect their sovereignty over their intellectual and cultural property.

Educate Others

Share the importance of cross-cultural respect with fellow herbalists, students, and enthusiasts. Encourage an environment of openness, curiosity, and appreciation for diverse herbal traditions.

Practice Ethical Wildcrafting

If engaged in wildcrafting or foraging, practice ethical and sustainable methods while respecting the ecosystems and cultural significance of the plants you harvest.

Be Mindful of Commercialization

Avoid commercialization that exploits cultural practices or sacred herbs for profit. Ensure that your herbal business practices are ethical and considerate of cultural sensitivities.

Connecting With Local Herbal Communities, Farms, and Shops

Building connections with local herbal communities, farms, and shops can be a rewarding and enriching experience for aspiring herbalists. These connections offer numerous benefits—from acquiring fresh, locally sourced herbs to gaining valuable knowledge and support. The benefits extend beyond acquiring herbs to include educational opportunities, community support, and a deeper connection to the natural world. Actively participating in local events and engaging with like-minded people will enrich your herbal journey and contribute to your local herbal community's network.

The Benefits of Connecting with Local Herbal Communities, Farms, and Shops

- **Access to fresh and local herbs**: Local herbal communities and farms often provide access to fresh, locally grown herbs, which can be more potent and flavorful than commercially sourced options.
- **Safer sources of herbs**: Local communities and establishments often aim to produce their herbs ecologically and without using harmful pesticides, thereby protecting the end-user from consuming residual chemicals with their herbs.
- **Educational opportunities**: Engaging with local herbalists and herbal communities can offer educational

opportunities, workshops, and classes to deepen your understanding of herbalism.

- **Networking and community support**: Connecting with local herbal communities fosters a sense of community. Networking with like-minded people provides support, encouragement, and opportunities for collaboration.
- **Seasonal awareness**: Local herbalists and farmers are attuned to the seasons, subsequently helping you understand the optimal times for harvesting specific herbs and promoting a connection with nature's cycles.
- **Sustainable and ethical sourcing**: Many local herbal farms prioritize sustainable and ethical growing practices allowing you to source herbs with a smaller ecological footprint.
- **Variety of herbal products**: Local herbal shops often offer a diverse range of herbal products—from teas and tinctures to salves and oils—providing a convenient and diverse selection.
- **Custom herbal blends**: Some local herbalists and shops offer the opportunity to create custom herbal blends tailored to your specific health needs and preferences.
- **Cultural and regional herbal wisdom**: Local herbal communities may possess unique cultural or regional herbal wisdom, thus, enriching your understanding of the diverse uses of plants.
- **Reduced carbon footprint**: Supporting local communities, farms, and shops reduces the carbon footprint of herb production by limiting the use of transport.

How to Connect with Local Herbal Communities, Farms, and Shops

- **Attend local events and workshops**: Look for herbal events, workshops, and classes in your area. Attend these gatherings to meet local herbalists and enthusiasts.
- **Join online platforms**: Participate in online forums, social media groups, or community websites focused on herbalism. This can help you discover local events and connect with herbalists in your region.
- **Visit farmers' markets**: Local farmers' markets often host herbalists and growers. Strike up conversations, ask questions, and express your interest in herbalism.
- **Community gardens**: Get involved in community gardens or herbal gardens in your neighborhood. This is an excellent way to meet people passionate about herbs and gardening.
- **Herb walks and nature tours**: Join guided herb walks or nature tours organized by local herbalists. This allows you to learn about local plants in their natural habitat.
- **Explore local herbal shops**: Visit local herbal shops, apothecaries, or health food stores that focus on herbal products. Strike up conversations with the staff to gain insights into the local herbal scene.
- **Volunteer at local farms**: Offer to volunteer at local herb farms or community gardens. This hands-on experience can deepen your knowledge and connect you with local growers.
- **Participate in community events**: Attend community events, fairs, or festivals that celebrate local produce and herbal products. These gatherings often attract local herbalists and farmers.
- **Ask for recommendations**: Seek recommendations from local health food stores, naturopaths, or alternative

health practitioners. They often have insights into the local herbal community, so you can track down local growers and suppliers.

- **Support local businesses**: Make a conscious effort to support local herbal businesses. Purchasing products from them not only makes community connections but also supports sustainable practices.

- **Create or join a local herbal meetup**: Consider starting or joining a local herbal meetup group. This can be a casual gathering where enthusiasts exchange knowledge, experiences, herbal remedies, and other herbal goods.

- **Participate in herbal Community Supported Agriculture (CSA) programs**: Some herbal farms offer CSA programs. Joining such programs provides you with access to a regular supply of fresh, locally-grown herbs.

Chapter 11

Global Herbal Traditions

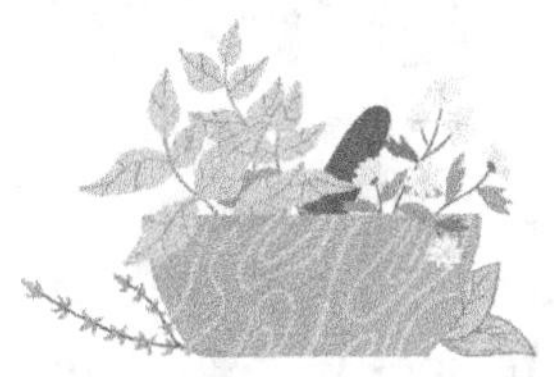

Introduction to the Global Spectrum of Herbal Traditions

The global spectrum of herbal traditions is a rich tapestry woven by diverse cultures around the world. Each culture has developed its unique approach to use plants for medicinal, spiritual, and culinary purposes. It is a testament to the diversity of human cultures and their deep relationships with plants. Exploring this spectrum reveals a fascinating array of practices, beliefs, and wisdom that span continents and centuries. As a budding herbalist, exploring this rich tapestry can provide valuable insights, broaden your perspective, and deepen your appreciation for the interconnected nature of herbal practices. Let us explore the global spectrum of herbal traditions:

Ayurveda (Indian Herbal Tradition)

A Brief History of Ayurveda

Ayurveda traces its roots to the Vedic period (1500–600 BCE) with early mentions in the Vedas—ancient Indian sacred texts.

The *Rigveda*, in particular, contains hymns praising the medicinal properties of various plants.

The *Charaka Samhita* and *Sushruta Samhita* (circa 6th century BCE) are the two foundational texts of Ayurveda. They comprehensively cover various aspects of medicine including anatomy, physiology, surgery, diagnosis, and the use of medicinal plants for healing.

Ayurveda flourished during the Buddhist period (6th–4th century BCE), subsequently gaining further recognition and influencing medicinal practices in regions where Buddhism spread.

The Gupta period (4th–6th century CE) saw significant developments in Ayurveda. The compilation of medical knowledge continued, and Ayurvedic practitioners gained patronage from rulers.

During the Islamic rule in India (8th–12th century), the exchange of knowledge between Ayurveda and Islamic medicine—known as Unani medicine—occurred. This period saw the synthesis of Ayurvedic and Persian medicinal traditions.

The colonial period (1858–1947) saw a decline in Ayurveda due to various factors including foreign influence, suppression of traditional practices, and the rise of Western medicine.

The late 20th century witnessed a resurgence of interest in Ayurveda driven by efforts to reclaim and revitalize India's traditional knowledge. Ayurveda gained official recognition and educational institutions were established.

25 Ayurvedic Herbs and Their Medicinal Uses

1. Amla, Amalaki, or Indian gooseberry (*Phyllanthus emblica*)

Parts used: whole plant

Medicinal uses:

- anti-aging
- stimulates hair growth
- immune system support
- regulates blood pressure and acidity
- wound healing

2. Arjuna (*Terminalia arjuna*)

Parts used: bark

Medicinal uses:

- reduces the risk of heart disease
- treatment of blood diseases, such as anemia and blood clots
- lowers blood pressure
- anti-inflammatory
- anti-carcinogenic

3. Ashwagandha or Indian ginseng (*Withania somnifera*)

Parts used: whole plant

Medicinal uses:

- anti-inflammatory
- lowers blood pressure
- reduces stress and anxiety

- treatment for insomnia
- immune system support

4. Bacopa, Brahmi, water hyssop (*Bacopa monnieri*)

Parts used: leaves, stems

Medicinal uses:

- anti-inflammatory
- antioxidant effects
- reduces stress and anxiety
- lowers blood pressure
- improves cognitive function

5. Borage or Mexican mint (*Borago officinalis*)

Parts used: flowers, leaves, seed oil

Medicinal uses:

- anti-inflammatory
- relieves symptoms of asthma
- treats skin conditions such as psoriasis, dermatitis, and eczema
- kidney support
- antidepressant effects

6. Bhringaraj or False Daisy (*Eclipta prostrata*)

Parts used: leaves, flowers

Medicinal uses:

- stimulates hair growth
- reduces dandruff
- helps prevent urinary tract infections

- treats skin conditions such as psoriasis, dermatitis, and eczema
- liver support

7. Boswellia, Indian frankincense, or olibanum (*Boswellia serrata*)

Parts used: gum resin

Medicinal uses:

- anti-inflammatory
- anticancer
- reduces pain associated with, osteoarthritis, rheumatoid arthritis, and inflammatory bowel disease
- decreased symptoms of asthma
- relieves symptoms of Parkinson's disease

8. Gotu kola, spadeleaf, or pennywort (*Centella asiatica*)

Parts used: leaves, stems

Medicinal uses:

- improves memory
- reduces stress and anxiety
- antidepressant effects
- improves circulation
- wound healing

9. Giloy, or Guduchi (*Tinospora cordifolia*)

Parts used: leaves, stems

Medicinal uses:

- immune system support

The Green Glow

- wound healing
- regulates blood sugar
- diarrhea
- gout

10. Guggul or Indian bdellium-tree (*Commiphora wightii*)

Parts used: gum resin

Medicinal uses:

- lowers cholesterol
- anti-Inflammatory
- treats skin conditions such as psoriasis, dermatitis, and eczema
- improves hyperthyroidism
- suppresses appetite

11. Hibiscus (*Hibiscus sabdariffa*)

Parts used: Whole plant

Medicinal uses:

- antioxidant effects
- lowers blood pressure
- lowers cholesterol
- liver support
- promotes weight loss

12. Milk Thistle (*Silybum marianum*)

Parts used: whole plant

Medicinal uses:

- liver support

- anti-inflammatory
- protects against bone loss
- regulates blood sugar
- prevents decline in brain function

13. Moringa or drumstick tree (*Moringa oleifera*)

Parts used: pods, leaves, flowers

Medicinal uses:

- antioxidant effects
- anti-inflammatory
- regulates blood sugar
- lowers cholesterol
- nutritional supplement

14. Macuna or Velvet Bean (*Mucuna pruriens*)

Parts used: beans

Medicinal uses:

- antidepressant effects
- nervous system support
- digestive aid
- improves coordination
- reproductive health support

15. Neem (*Azadirachta indica*)

Parts used: whole plant

Medicinal uses:

- immune system support
- prevent skin problems

The Green Glow

- regulates blood sugar
- digestive aid
- wound healing

16. Punarnava or Spreading Hogsweed (*Boerhaavia diffusa*)

Parts used: whole plant

Medicinal uses:

- kidney support
- liver support
- promotes weight loss
- helps prevent urinary tract infections
- relieves symptoms of nephritic syndrome

17. Sesame (*Sesamum indicum*)

Parts used: seeds, seed oil, leaves

Medicinal uses:

- anti-inflammatory
- heart health support
- regulates blood sugar
- relieves symptoms of arthritis
- wound healing

18. Shatavari (*Asparagus racemosus*)

Parts used: roots

Medicinal uses:

- improves female reproductive health
- reduces anxiety
- improves lactation in breast-feeding women

- digestive aid
- hormone regulation

19. Tulsi or Holy Basil (*Ocimum sanctum*)

Parts used: leaves, stems, flowers, seeds

Medicinal uses:

- reduces stress and anxiety
- antioxidant effects
- anti-inflammatory
- wound healing
- regulates blood sugar

20. Turmeric (*Curcuma longa*)

Parts used: rhizomes

Medicinal uses:

- anti-inflammatory
- helps prevent heart disease
- anticancer
- antidepressant effects
- helps treat Alzheimer's disease

21. Manjistha or Indian Madder (*Rubia cordifolia*)

Parts used: roots, stems

Medicinal uses:

- treats calcium deficiency
- treats skin conditions such as psoriasis, dermatitis, and eczema
- relieves menstrual pain

The Green Glow

- anticancer
- detoxifying effects

22. Pippali or Long Pepper (*Piper longum*)

Parts used: roots, fruits

Medicinal uses:

- antidepressant effects
- antioxidant effects
- immune system support
- reduces stress and anxiety
- relieves symptoms of Parkinson's disease

23. Vasaka or Malabar Nut (*Adhatoda vasica*)

Parts used: whole plant

Medicinal uses:

- anti-inflammatory
- decongestant
- relieves symptoms of asthma
- wound healing
- antioxidant effects

24. Shardunika or Australian Cowplant (*Gymnema sylvestre*)

Parts used: leaves, roots

Medicinal uses:

- regulates blood sugar
- reduces sugar cravings
- reduces cholesterol
- promotes weight loss

- anti-inflammatory

25. Kalmegh or King of the Bitters (*Andrographis paniculata*)

Parts used: whole plant

Medicinal uses:

- immune system support
- liver support
- digestive aid
- anti-inflammatory
- anti-microbial

Traditional Chinese Medicine

A Brief History of Traditional Chinese Medicine

Attributed to the legendary Yellow Emperor, the Huangdi Neijing (475–221 BCE) is a seminal text that lays the foundation for TCM. It discusses Yin and Yang, the Five Elements, and the flow of Qi (vital energy).

Shanghan Lun, authored by Zhang Zhongjing (220–420 CE), delves into the diagnosis and treatment of febrile diseases. It introduces the concept of syndromes and patterns, consequently laying the groundwork for clinical practice.

The Tang Dynasty (618–907) witnessed the establishment of the Imperial Medical College. Developments in acupuncture and herbal medicine continued, and medical texts were compiled.

The Song Dynasty (960–1279) saw advancements in medical knowledge. Notable figures like Sun Simiao contributed to herbal medicine, and pulse diagnosis became more refined.

The Green Glow

During the Ming and Qing dynasties (1368–1912), TCM theories were further consolidated. The *Compendium of Materia Medica* by Li Shizhen documented thousands of herbs and their medicinal uses.

The 20th century posed challenges to TCM as Western medicine gained prominence. TCM faced criticism, and efforts were made to modernize its practices.

The Cultural Revolution had a significant impact on TCM. Traditional practices were suppressed, and many practitioners faced persecution.

In the latter half of the 20th century, there was a revival of interest in TCM. The Chinese government recognized its value, and efforts were made to integrate TCM with Western medicine.

Today, TCM is integrated into the Chinese healthcare system, and there is ongoing research to validate its efficacy. It coexists with Western medicine, providing patients with a range of treatment options.

25 TCM Herbs and Their Uses

1. Korean Mint (*Agastache rugosa*)

Parts used: leaves, stems

Medicinal uses:

- respiratory support
- reduces nausea
- calming effect
- digestive aid
- anti-inflammatory

2. Chinese Alangium (*Alangium chinense*)

Parts used: whole plant

Medicinal uses:

- wound healing
- anti-inflammatory
- pain relief
- digestive aid
- liver Support

3. Japanese Ardisia or Marlberry (*Ardisia japonica*)

Parts used: leaves, stems

Medicinal uses:

- expectorant
- anticancer
- stimulates blood circulation
- detoxifying effect
- relieves bloating and flatulence

4. Tatarian Aster (*Aster tataricus*)

Parts used: leaves, roots

Medicinal uses:

- reducing stomach acid
- reduces nausea
- anti-inflammatory
- respiratory support
- digestive support

5. Tea Plant (*Camellia sinensis*)

Parts used: leaves, stems

Medicinal uses:

- protecting the skin from UV radiation
- heart health
- anticancer
- immune system support
- calming effect

6. Safflower (*Carthamus tinctorius*)

Parts used: flowers, seeds, oil

Medicinal uses:

- cardiovascular health
- wound healing
- weight loss
- regulates blood sugar
- menstrual health

7. Velvet Leaf (*Cissampelos pareira*)

Parts used: whole plant

Medicinal uses:

- anti-inflammatory
- fever reduction
- rheumatism
- respiratory support
- digestive disorders

8. Yan Hu Suo (*Corydalis yanhusuo*)

Parts used: rhizomes

Medicinal uses:

- pain relief
- menstrual disorders
- cardiovascular health
- anti-inflammatory
- mood enhancement

9. Lilac Daphne (*Daphne genkwa*)

Parts used: flowers

Medicinal uses:

- anti-inflammatory
- respiratory support
- antimicrobial
- treats skin conditions such as psoriasis, dermatitis, and eczema
- rheumatism

10. Noble Rock Orchid (*Dendrobium nobile*)

Parts used: stems, leaves

Medicinal uses:

- anti-aging
- immune system support
- improves digestion
- anti-inflammatory
- lowers blood pressure

11. Blue Evergreen Hydrangea (*Dichroa febrifuga*)

Parts used: root, bark

Medicinal uses:

- anti-inflammatory
- fever reduction
- rheumatism
- treatment for malaria
- respiratory support

12. Hardy Rubber Tree (*Eucommia ulmoides*)

Parts used: bark, leaves

Medicinal uses:

- blood pressure regulation
- anti-inflammatory
- bone health
- adrenal support
- anti-aging

13. Bushweed (Flueggea suffruticosa)

Parts used: whole plant

Medicinal uses:

- anti-inflammatory
- fever reduction
- analgesic
- skin conditions
- respiratory issues

14. Loureiro's Gentian (*Gentiana loureiroi*)

Parts used: roots

Medicinal uses:

- digestive aid
- bitter tonic
- anti-inflammatory
- liver support
- fever reduction

15. Chinese Licorice (*Glycyrrhiza uralensis*)

Parts used: root

Medicinal uses:

- anti-inflammatory
- cough and cold
- adrenal support
- gastric ulcers
- immune system support

16. Purple Holly (*Ilex purpurea*)

Parts used: leaves

Medicinal uses:

- diuretic
- anti-inflammatory
- circulatory support
- digestive aid
- antioxidant

17. Chinese Lovage (*Ligusticum wallichii*)

Parts used: root

Medicinal uses:

- menstrual disorders
- blood circulation
- anti-inflammatory
- pain relief
- respiratory support

18. Amur Cork Tree (*Phellodendron amurense*)

Parts used: bark

Medicinal uses:

- anti-inflammatory
- antioxidant
- immune system support
- digestive health
- skin conditions

19. Golden Larch (*Pseudolarix amabilis*)

Parts used: resin

Medicinal uses:

- antimicrobial
- anti-inflammatory
- wound healing
- respiratory health
- arthritis

20. Kudzu (*Pueraria lobata*)

Parts used: root

Medicinal uses:

- alcoholism treatment
- cardiovascular health
- menopausal symptoms
- blood sugar control
- anti-inflammatory

21. Chinese Foxglove (*Rehmannia glutinosa*)

Parts used: root

Medicinal uses:

- adrenal support
- kidney health
- anti-inflammatory
- liver health
- blood tonic

22. Qinghai Rhododendron (*Rhododendron qinghaiense*)

Parts used: whole plant

Medicinal uses:

- anti-inflammatory
- fever reduction
- respiratory conditions
- skin disorders
- antioxidant

23. Chinese Magnolia Vine (*Schisandra chinensis*)

Parts used: berries, seeds

Medicinal uses:

- adaptogenic properties
- liver health
- anti-inflammatory
- stress relief
- respiratory health

24. Indian Sarsaparilla (*Stemona tuberosa*)

Parts used: roots

Medicinal uses:

- respiratory health
- antimicrobial
- skin disorders
- expectorant
- anti-inflammatory

25. Japanese Pagoda Tree (*Styphnolobium japonicum*)

Parts used: bark, flowers

Medicinal uses:

- anti-Inflammatory
- antioxidant effects
- bone health
- respiratory health
- cardiovascular support

African Traditional Medicine

A Brief History of African Traditional Medicine

African traditional medicine (ATM) is a diverse and ancient system of healing that has been practiced on the continent for thousands of years. Rooted in the cultural and spiritual beliefs of diverse African societies, ATM encompasses a holistic approach to health and well-being. Great Zimbabwe—a medieval kingdom —and the Swahili Coast witnessed the development of trade routes facilitating the exchange of medicinal knowledge between different regions.

Ancient Egypt contributed to early medical knowledge. Papyri such as the Ebers Papyrus contained medicinal recipes and surgical techniques.

Indigenous African communities have practiced traditional healing for millennia. Traditional healers often served as inter-mediaries between the physical and spiritual realms. Ancestor worship and the acknowledgment of spiritual forces were central to healing rituals. Healing rituals and ceremonies were integral to traditional medicine. These events were not only therapeutic but served to restore balance within the person themselves as well as the community.

Traditional healers possessed extensive knowledge of herbs and their applications often transmitted orally through griots, story-tellers, or respected elders. This ensured the continuity of healing wisdom across generations.

The colonial era brought significant challenges to ATM. Western powers often marginalized and undermined traditional healing practices while favoring Western medical approaches. Missionary activities further contributed to the stigmatization of traditional healing branding it as "pagan" or "superstitious."

With the wave of independence movements in the mid 20th century, there was a renewed interest in reclaiming and preserving African cultural practices including traditional medicine. Many African countries have taken steps to recognize and integrate traditional medicine into their healthcare systems. National policies have been developed to support the coexistence of traditional and Western medical practices.

ATM is now recognized as a valuable component of healthcare in many African countries. Efforts have been made to integrate traditional healers into formal healthcare systems.

25 African Traditional Medicine Herbs and Their Uses

1. Baobab (*Adansonia digitata*)

Parts used: fruit pulp, leaves, bark, seeds

Medicinal uses:

- antioxidant effects
- digestive health
- source of vitamin C
- anti-inflammatory
- relieves symptoms of dehydration

2. Krantz Aloe (*Aloe arborescens*)

Parts used: leaves (gel and latex)

Medicinal uses:

- skin health
- digestive aid
- immune system boost
- anti-inflammatory
- antioxidant properties

3. Cashew (*Anacardium occidentale*)

Parts used: nuts, leaves

Medicinal uses:

- heart health
- anti-inflammatory
- bone health
- anti-diabetic
- weight management

4. African Wormwood (*Artemisia afra*)

Parts used: leaves

Medicinal uses:

- digestive health
- malaria treatment
- anti-inflammatory
- respiratory conditions
- antibacterial

5. Wild Cucumber (*Cucumis africanus*)

Parts used: fruit, seeds

Medicinal uses:

- hydration
- skin conditions
- kidney health
- detoxification
- anti-inflammatory

6. Rhino Bush (*Ellytropappus rhinocerotis*)

Parts used: whole plant

Medicinal uses:

- digestive aid
- respiratory conditions
- fever reduction
- anti-inflammatory
- antioxidant properties

7. Pale Yellow Eriosema (*Eriosema kraussianum*)

Parts used: whole plant

Medicinal uses:

- reproductive health
- anti-inflammatory
- urinary disorders
- fever reduction
- wound healing

8. Corn Lily (*Gladiolus dalenii*)

Parts used: corms, stems

Medicinal uses:

- menopause
- anti-inflammatory
- pain relief
- digestive disorders
- fever reduction

9. Devil's Claw (*Harpagophytum procumbens*)

Parts used: roots, tubers

Medicinal uses:

- arthritis
- pain relief
- digestive issues
- anti-inflammatory
- fever reduction

10. Curry Plant or Italian Strawflower (*Helichrysum species*)

Parts used: leaves, flowers

Medicinal uses:

- anti-inflammatory
- antioxidant properties
- skin health
- respiratory health
- wound healing

11. Sausage Tree (*Kigelia africana*)

Parts used: fruit, bark, leaves

Medicinal uses:

- skin conditions
- anti-inflammatory
- breast firming
- antibacterial
- immune system support

12. Balsam Pear (*Momordica balsamina L.*)

Parts used: fruits, leaves

Medicinal uses:

- blood sugar control
- digestive health
- anti-inflammatory
- antioxidant properties
- wound healing

13. African Geranium (*Pelargonium sidoides*)

Parts used: roots

Medicinal uses:

- respiratory conditions
- cough and cold
- immune system support
- antibacterial
- bronchitis

14. Scurfy Pea (*Psoralea pinnata*)

Parts used: whole plant

Medicinal uses:

- emotional stress relief
- skin disorders
- anti-inflammatory
- fever reduction
- urinary disorders

15. Kanna (*Sceletium tortuosum*)

Parts used: leaves, stems

Medicinal uses:

- mood enhancement
- anxiety and depression
- cognitive function
- appetite suppressant
- pain relief

16. African Ginger (*Siphonochilus aethiopicus*)

Parts used: rhizomes

Medicinal uses:

- digestive health
- anti-inflammatory
- antioxidant effects
- respiratory conditions
- fever reduction

17. Cancer Bush (*Sutherlandia frutescens*)

Parts used: leaves, stems

Medicinal uses:

- immune system support
- anticancer properties
- diabetes management
- liver health
- anti-inflammatory

18. Wild Garlic (*Tulbaghia violacea*)

Parts used: bulbs, leaves

Medicinal uses:

- antibacterial
- cardiovascular health
- respiratory conditions
- digestive health
- anti-inflammatory

19. Pepper-Bark Tree (*Warburgia salutaris*)

Parts used: bark, leaves

Medicinal uses:

- antibacterial
- respiratory health
- digestive health
- anti-inflammatory
- fever reduction

20. Madagascar Periwinkle (*Catharanthus roseus*)

Parts used: leaves, flowers

Medicinal uses:

- anti-cancer
- diabetes management
- blood pressure
- anti-microbial
- circulatory health

21. African Black Bean (*Griffonia simplicifolia*)

Parts used: seeds

Medicinal uses:

- serotonin regulation
- anxiety and depression
- sleep aid
- appetite suppressant
- migraine relief

22. Climbing Oleander (*Strophanthus gratus*)

Parts used: seeds

Medicinal uses:

- cardiovascular health
- anti-inflammatory
- analgesic
- respiratory conditions
- muscle relaxant

23. Rosary Pea (*Abrus precatorius*)

Parts used: seeds

Medicinal uses:

- fever reduction
- anti-inflammatory
- pain relief
- anti-cancer
- abortifacient

24. Soursop (*Annona muricata*)

Parts used: leaves, fruit, seeds

Medicinal uses:

- anti-cancer
- digestive health
- immune system support
- anti-inflammatory
- antioxidant properties

25. Hairy Spurge (*Euphorbia hirta*)

Parts used: whole plant

Medicinal uses:

- respiratory health
- asthma relief
- anti-inflammatory
- skin disorders
- diuretic

Native American Herbalism

A Brief History of Native American Herbalism

Native American herbalism is a rich and intricate system of healing that has been woven into the fabric of indigenous cultures across North and South America for thousands of years. Rooted in a deep connection with the land, plants, and spiritual beliefs, Native American herbalism reflects a holistic approach to health.

Native American tribes had profound connections to their environments. The land provided not only sustenance but also the foundation for spiritual and medicinal practices.

Knowledge of herbal medicine was transmitted orally from generation to generation. Elders and medicine men and women played crucial roles as wisdom keepers, passing down the sacred knowledge of plants.

Many plants held medicinal and spiritual qualities to Native American herbalists, who often integrated healing practices with spiritual ceremonies.

Trade networks facilitated the exchange of plant knowledge among tribes. Different regions benefited from the wisdom of plants that were not native to their immediate surroundings.

The arrival of European settlers brought profound challenges to Native American herbalism. Native practices were often suppressed, and traditional healers faced persecution. Despite the challenges, many Native American communities worked tirelessly to preserve their herbal traditions. Secretive practices and underground preservation efforts helped safeguard the sacred knowledge. The latter half of the 20th century witnessed a cultural renaissance within Native American communities. Efforts were made to revitalize and share traditional practices, including herbalism.

In recent years, there has been an increased recognition of the value of traditional Native American herbalism. Legal protections have been established to respect and preserve indigenous knowledge.

25 Herbs Used in Native American Herbalism and Their Uses

1. Barberry (*Berberis genus*)

Parts used: bark, root, berries

Medicinal uses:

- digestive health
- antibacterial
- liver health
- heart health
- immune system support

2. Candle Bush (*Cassia alata*)

Parts used: Leaves, flowers

Medicinal uses:

- antifungal
- skin conditions
- anti-inflammatory
- antibacterial
- detoxifying effects

3. Horsemint (*Monarda genus*)

Parts used: leaves, flowers

Medicinal uses:

- antiseptic
- digestive aid
- respiratory health
- anti-inflammatory
- headache relief

4. Cascara Buckthorn (*Rhamnus purshiana*)

Parts used: bark

Medicinal uses:

- laxative
- digestive health
- liver health
- constipation relief
- colon cleansing

5. Cinchona (*Cinchona sp.*)

Parts used: bark

Medicinal uses:

- antimalarial
- fever reduction
- digestive health
- muscle relaxant
- anti-inflammatory

6. Juniper (*Juniperus sp.*)

Parts used: berries, essential oil

Medicinal uses:

- diuretic
- joint pain
- respiratory health
- antibacterial
- digestive aid

7. Willow (*Salix sp.*)

Parts used: bark, leaves

Medicinal uses:

- pain relief
- anti-inflammatory
- fever reduction
- headache relief
- arthritis

8. Dogwood (*Cornus florida*)

Parts used: bark

Medicinal uses:

- anti-inflammatory
- fever reduction
- urinary disorders
- skin conditions
- respiratory health

9. Geranium (*Geranium sp.*)

Parts used: leaves, flowers

Medicinal uses:

- astringent
- wound healing
- anti-inflammatory
- diarrhea relief
- skin health

10. Ginseng (*Panax quinquefolium*)

Parts used: roots

Medicinal uses:

- adaptogen
- energy boost
- immune system support
- cognitive function
- anti-inflammatory

11. Wormseed (*Chenopodium ambrosioides*)

Parts used: leaves, seeds

Medicinal uses:

- antiparasitic
- digestive health
- fever reduction
- respiratory health
- skin conditions

12. White Hellebore (*Veratrum viride*)

Parts used: rhizomes

Medicinal uses:

- hypertension
- antiarrhythmic
- antispasmodic
- diaphoretic
- nausea and vomiting

13. Greek Valerian (*Polemonium reptans*)

Parts used: roots

Medicinal uses:

- relaxant
- anxiety relief
- cough and cold
- fever reduction
- sleep aid

14. Elderberry (*Sambucus canadensis*)

Parts used: berries, flowers

Medicinal uses:

- immune system support
- antiviral
- respiratory health
- anti-inflammatory
- cold and flu relief

15. Angelica (*Angelica atropurpurea*)

Parts used: roots, stems

Medicinal uses:

- digestive aid
- anti-inflammatory
- respiratory health
- menstrual disorders
- diuretic

16. Witch Hazel (*Hamamelis virginiana*)

Parts used: bark, leaves

Medicinal uses:

- astringent
- anti-inflammatory
- skin conditions
- hemorrhoids
- minor wounds

17. Pipsissewa (*Chimaphila umbellata*)

Parts used: leaves

Medicinal uses:

- diuretic
- urinary disorders
- kidney health
- anti-inflammatory
- rheumatism

18. Balsam Fir (*Abies balsamea*)

Parts used: resin, needles

Medicinal uses:

- respiratory health
- anti-inflammatory
- wound healing
- joint pain
- cough and cold

19. Arrowwood (*Viburnum dentatum*)

Parts used: bark

Medicinal uses:

- antispasmodic
- menstrual disorders
- uterine tonic
- fever reduction
- pain relief

20. Bloodroot (*Sanguinaria canadensis*)

Parts used: rhizomes, sap

Medicinal uses:

- skin conditions
- respiratory health
- antimicrobial
- digestive aid
- anti-inflammatory

21. Yucca (*Yucca elata Englemann*)

Parts used: roots

Medicinal uses:

- joint health
- anti-inflammatory
- digestive aid
- skin conditions
- antioxidant properties

22. Mescal or Agave (*Agave parryi*)

Parts used: sap (agave syrup)

Medicinal uses:

- sweetener
- wound healing
- anti-inflammatory
- digestive health
- skin conditions

23. Mesquite (*Prosopis glandulosa*)

Parts used: pods, seeds

Medicinal uses:

- digestive health
- blood sugar regulation
- antioxidant properties
- respiratory health
- nutrient source

24. Bitterroot (*Acorus calamus*)

Parts used: rhizomes

Medicinal uses:

- digestive aid
- mental clarity
- anti-inflammatory
- respiratory health
- aphrodisiac

25. Osha (*Ligusticum porter*)

Parts used: roots

Medicinal uses:

- respiratory health
- cough and cold
- antiviral
- immune system support
- fever reduction

European Herbalism

A Brief History of European Herbalism

European herbalism is deeply interwoven with the continent's history, spanning thousands of years and evolving through diverse cultures.

The ancient Greeks, particularly Hippocrates (460–370 BCE), contributed significantly to the foundations of Western herbalism. The Hippocratic Corpus, a collection of medical texts, emphasized the use of herbs in maintaining balance within the body. Pedanius Dioscorides, a Greek physician, wrote *De Materia Medica* in the 1st century CE. This comprehensive herbal guide described hundreds of medicinal plants and influenced European herbalism for centuries. Galen, a prominent Roman physician (129—210), further developed the principles of Greek medicine. His humoral theory and medicinal plant knowledge became integral to European herbal traditions.

During the Middle Ages, monasteries played a central role in preserving and expanding herbal knowledge. Monks cultivated gardens containing medicinal plants, and monastic herbalism became a cornerstone of healthcare.

Hildegard of Bingen (1098–1179), a German abbess, contributed significantly to herbal medicine. Her work, *Physica*, discussed the healing properties of plants and emphasized their connection to divine creation.

The Renaissance saw a revival of interest in classical Greek and Roman texts, including those on herbalism. Scholars rediscovered and translated ancient works, contributing to the wealth of herbal knowledge.

The herbal Renaissance in the 16th and 17th centuries involved the publication of herbal texts, botanical illustrations, and the establishment of herbal gardens. Notable works include John Gerard's *Herball* and Nicholas Culpeper's *Complete Herbal*.

Carl Linnaeus (1707–1778) introduced systematic botanical classification, providing a scientific framework for studying plants. His work laid the foundation for modern botany and herbalism.

The 19th century witnessed the impact of industrialization on herbalism. Traditional practices coexisted with the rise of pharmaceuticals, leading to a shift in healthcare approaches.

The late 20th and early 21st centuries have seen a revival of interest in herbalism. People are rediscovering the value of natural remedies, and herbal practices are integrated into complementary and alternative medicine.

25 Herbs Used in European Herbalism and Their Uses

1. European Blackberry (*Rubus fruticosus*)

Parts used: berries, leaves, roots

Medicinal uses:

- antioxidant
- digestive health

- anti-inflammatory
- immune system support
- oral health

2. Verbena (*Verbena officinalis*)

Parts used: leaves, flowers

Medicinal uses:

- calms the nerves
- digestive aid
- respiratory health
- anti-inflammatory
- sleep aid

3. Agrimony (*Agrimonia eupatoria*)

Parts used: leaves, flowers

Medicinal uses:

- astringent
- digestive health
- wound healing
- anti-inflammatory
- liver health

4. Henbane (*Hyoscyamus niger*)

Parts used: leaves, seeds

Medicinal uses:

- analgesic
- sedative
- antispasmodic

* respiratory health
* topical pain relief

5. Ribwort Plantain (*Plantago lanceolata*)

Parts used: leaves, seeds

Medicinal uses:

* demulcent
* anti-inflammatory
* wound healing
* respiratory health
* digestive aid

6. Poppy (*Papaver somniferum*)

Parts used: seeds, latex (opium)

Medicinal uses:

* analgesic
* cough suppressant
* sleep aid
* antidiarrheal
* anxiolytic

7. Wild Strawberry (*Fragaria vesca*)

Parts used: leaves, berries

Medicinal uses:

* antioxidant
* digestive health
* anti-inflammatory
* skin conditions

The Green Glow

- urinary health

8. Meadowsweet (*Filipendula ulmaria*)

Parts used: flowers, leaves

Medicinal uses:

- anti-inflammatory
- digestive aid
- pain relief
- fever reduction
- respiratory health

9. Gromwell (*Lithospermum purpurocaeruleum*)

Parts used: roots

Medicinal uses:

- anti-inflammatory
- skin conditions
- wound healing
- respiratory health
- urinary health

10. Pigweed (*Chenopodium album*)

Parts used: leaves, seeds

Medicinal uses:

- antioxidant
- anti-inflammatory
- digestive aid
- nutrient source
- antiseptic

11. Hazelnut (*Corylus sp.*)

Parts used: nuts, bark

Medicinal uses:

- cardiovascular health
- anti-inflammatory
- skin conditions
- digestive health
- nutrient source

12. Crab Apple (*Malus sp.*)

Parts used: fruit, bark

Medicinal uses:

- digestive aid
- antioxidant
- skin conditions
- cardiovascular health
- liver health

13. Stinging Nettle (*Urtica dioica*)

Parts used: leaves, roots

Medicinal uses:

- anti-inflammatory
- allergies
- diuretic
- joint health
- nutrient source

14. Hemlock (*Conium maculatum*)

Parts used: whole plant

Medicinal uses:

- analgesic
- sedative
- muscle relaxant
- respiratory health
- topical pain relief

15. White Violet (*Viola alba*)

Parts used: flowers, leaves

Medicinal uses:

- anti-inflammatory
- skin conditions
- respiratory health
- cough suppressant
- diuretic

16. Broadleaf Plantain (*Plantago major*)

Parts used: leaves, seeds

Medicinal uses:

- demulcent
- anti-inflammatory
- wound healing
- digestive aid
- respiratory health

17. Celery (*Apium graveolens*)

Parts used: stems, seeds

Medicinal uses:

- anti-inflammatory
- digestive aid
- blood pressure
- diuretic
- joint health

18. Camelina (*Camelina sativa*)

Parts used: seeds

Medicinal uses:

- anti-inflammatory
- skin conditions
- cardiovascular health
- joint health
- nutrient source

19. Parsley (*Petroselinum crispum*)

Parts used: leaves, seeds

Medicinal uses:

- digestive aid
- diuretic
- antioxidant
- anti-inflammatory
- nutrient source

20. Hazel (*Corylus avellana*)

Parts used: leaves, bark

Medicinal uses:

- anti-inflammatory
- digestive health
- skin conditions
- respiratory health
- joint health

21. Dyer's Weed (*Reseda luteola*)

Parts used: leaves, flowers

Medicinal uses:

- anti-inflammatory
- skin conditions
- respiratory health
- liver health
- digestive aid

22. Black Pepper (*Piper nigrum*)

Parts used: fruits (peppercorns)

Medicinal uses:

- digestive aid
- anti-inflammatory
- antioxidant
- respiratory health
- cognitive function

23. Nutmeg (*Myristica fragrans*)

Parts used: seeds

Medicinal uses:

- digestive aid
- anti-inflammatory
- pain relief
- sleep aid
- mood enhancement

24. Celtic Nard (*Valeriana celtica*)

Parts used: rhizomes, roots

Medicinal uses:

- sedative
- sleep aid
- anxiety relief
- digestive aid
- muscle relaxant

25. Wormwood (*Artemisia absinthium*)

Parts used: leaves, flowers

Medicinal uses:

- digestive aid
- parasitic infections
- malaria
- anti-inflammatory
- fever reduction

Herbal Remedies Across Lesser-Known Traditions

Tibetan Medicine

Tibetan Medicine, also known as Sowa Rigpa, is an ancient healing system that originated in Tibet. It has strong roots in indigenous Tibetan practices, Ayurveda, and Chinese medicine.

Grounded in Buddhist principles, it emphasizes the balance of the three fundamental energies or humors—wind (rlung), bile (mKhris-pa), and phlegm (Bad-kan).

Tibetan Medicine uses a variety of unique herbs found in the Himalayan region such as Himalayan Rhubarb, Muskroot, and Himalayan Mayapple.

The system addresses a wide range of health issues, including digestive disorders, respiratory conditions, mental health, and spiritual well-being.

Kampo (Japanese Herbalism)

Kampo is a traditional Japanese herbal medicine system that originated from Chinese medicine but has evolved with unique Japanese influences.

The practice revolves around balancing the body's vital energy (Qi) and incorporates principles of Yin and Yang. Kampo emphasizes the importance of individualized treatments.

Kampo is applied to address a wide range of health concerns including digestive issues, respiratory conditions, and immune system support.

Unani Medicine

Unani Medicine, also known as Greco-Arabic medicine, has its roots in ancient Greek and Roman medicine and further developed in the Islamic world, particularly during the Golden Age of Islam.

Unani emphasizes the balance of the four humors for health: Dam—blood, Balgham—phlegm, Sauda—black bile, and Safra —yellow bile.

Unani Medicine takes a holistic approach, addressing various health issues related to digestion, respiratory health, and overall well-being.

Persian Herbalism

Persian Herbalism has a rich history rooted in ancient Persian and Islamic traditions. It incorporates influences from Zoroastrian and Islamic teachings.

Emphasizes maintaining balance and harmony within the body. It has a holistic approach to health and wellness.

Persian herbalism addresses a variety of health issues including digestive problems, respiratory conditions, and nervous system support.

25 Herbs From These Lesser-Known Traditions

1. Chervil (*Anthriscus cerefolium*)

Tradition: Tibetan medicine

Parts used: leaves, stems

Medicinal uses:

- diuretic
- digestive aid
- lowers blood pressure
- gout
- expectorant

2. Jujube (*Ziziphus jujuba*)

Tradition: Kampo

Parts used: fruits

Medicinal uses:

- calming the mind
- improving digestion
- immune system support
- stress reduction
- liver health

3. Black Seed (*Nigella sativa*)

Tradition: Unani medicine

Parts used: seeds

Medicinal uses:

- immune system booster
- anti-inflammatory
- respiratory health
- digestive aid
- antioxidant

4. Golpar (*Heracleum persicum*)

Tradition: Persian herbalism

Parts used: seeds

Medicinal uses:

- digestive aid
- anti-inflammatory

- respiratory health
- cardiovascular support
- antispasmodic

5. Himalayan Rhubarb (*Rheum emodi*)

Tradition: Tibetan medicine

Parts used: rhizomes

Medicinal uses:

- digestive health
- liver support
- laxative
- anti-inflammatory
- detoxification

6. Licorice Fern (*Polypodium glycyrrhiza*)

Tradition: Kampo

Parts used: rhizomes

Medicinal uses:

- immune system support
- respiratory health
- anti-inflammatory
- digestive aid
- adaptogen

7. Costus Root (*Saussurea lappa*)

Tradition: Unani medicine

Parts used: rhizomes

The Green Glow

Medicinal uses:

- respiratory health
- digestive aid
- anti-inflammatory
- antispasmodic
- immune system support

8. Asafoetida (*Ferula assa-foetida*)

Tradition: Persian herbalism

Parts used: resin (gum)

Medicinal uses:

- digestive aid
- respiratory health
- anti-inflammatory
- calms the nerves
- antispasmodic

9. Indian Valerian (*Valeriana wallichii*)

Tradition: Tibetan medicine

Parts used: rhizomes, roots

Medicinal uses:

- calms the nerves
- sleep aid
- stress reduction
- antispasmodic
- muscle relaxant

10. Japanese Honeysuckle (*Lonicera japonica*)

Tradition: Kampo

Parts used: flowers, stems

Medicinal uses:

- anti-inflammatory
- immune system support
- respiratory health
- antiviral
- detoxification

11. Myrrh (*Commiphora spp.*)

Tradition: Unani medicine

Parts used: resin (gum)

Medicinal uses:

- anti-inflammatory
- respiratory health
- antimicrobial
- wound healing
- immune system support

12. Saffron (*Crocus sativus*)

Tradition: Persian herbalism

Parts used: stigmas

Medicinal uses:

- antidepressant
- digestive aid

The Green Glow

- anti-inflammatory
- cardiovascular support
- immune system support

13. Himalayan Birch (*Betula utilis*)

Tradition: Tibetan medicine

Parts used: bark, leaves

Medicinal uses:

- anti-inflammatory
- analgesic (pain relief)
- respiratory health
- immune system support
- fever reduction

14. Japanese Knotweed (*Polygonum cuspidatum*)

Tradition: Kampo

Parts used: rhizomes

Medicinal uses:

- anti-inflammatory
- cardiovascular support
- antioxidant
- joint health
- antimicrobial

15. Belleric Myrobalan (*Terminalia bellirica*)

Tradition: Unani medicine

Parts used: fruits

Medicinal uses:

- digestive aid
- respiratory health
- liver support
- antioxidant
- laxative

16. Turmeric Sagebrush (*Artemisia sieversiana*)

Tradition: Tibetan medicine

Parts used: leaves

Medicinal uses:

- digestive aid
- anti-inflammatory
- respiratory health
- antioxidant
- antimicrobial

17. Japanese Clematis (*Clematis terniflora*)

Tradition: Kampo

Parts used: roots, stems

Medicinal uses:

- anti-inflammatory
- analgesic (pain relief)
- joint health
- immune system support
- antispasmodic

18. Muskroot (*Ferula moschata*)

Tradition: Unani medicine

Parts used: resin (gum)

Medicinal uses:

- calms the nerves
- aphrodisiac
- digestive aid
- antispasmodic
- respiratory health

19. Galangal (*Alpinia galanga*)

Tradition: Persian herbalism

Parts used: rhizomes

Medicinal uses:

- digestive aid
- anti-inflammatory
- respiratory health
- antioxidant
- aphrodisiac

20. Himalayan Mayapple (*Podophyllum hexandrum*)

Tradition: Tibetan medicine

Parts used: rhizomes

Medicinal uses:

- antiviral
- digestive aid

- immune system support
- liver support
- antioxidant

21. Chinese Skullcap (*Scutellaria baicalensis*)

Tradition: Kampo

Parts used: roots

Medicinal uses:

- anti-inflammatory
- calms the nerves
- antiviral
- respiratory health
- liver support

22. Arabian Olibanum (*Boswellia sacra*)

Tradition: Unani medicine

Parts used: resin (gum)

Medicinal uses:

- anti-inflammatory
- respiratory health
- wound healing
- immune system support
- calms the nerves

23. Purple Mint (*Mentha longifolia*)

Tradition: Persian herbalism

Parts used: leaves

The Green Glow

Medicinal uses:

- digestive aid
- respiratory health
- calms the nerves
- antispasmodic
- headache relief

24. Himalayan Teasel (*Dipsacus inermis*)

Tradition: Tibetan medicine

Parts used: roots

Medicinal uses:

- joint health
- anti-inflammatory
- analgesic (pain relief)
- immune system support
- digestive aid

25. Japanese Persimmon (*Diospyros kaki*)

Tradition: Kampo

Parts used: fruits

Medicinal uses:

- digestive aid
- cardiovascular support
- antioxidant
- respiratory health
- immune system support

Chapter 12

The Lifelong Journey Ahead

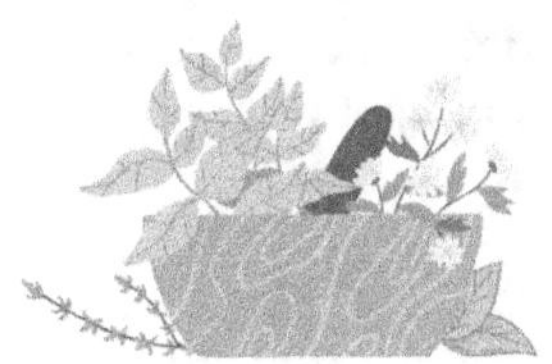

Embracing the Holistic and Interconnected Nature of Herbalism

Herbalism is more than a collection of remedies; it is a holistic approach to health that acknowledges the interconnectedness of the body, mind, and the natural world. Embracing the holistic and interconnected nature of herbalism involves recognizing the profound relationships between humans and plants, understanding the mind-body connection, and appreciating the ecological impact of herbal practices. Through this lens, herbalism transcends the idea of isolated remedies and becomes a lifestyle that nourishes not only the body but also the soul and the ecosystem we are part of.

Holistic Approach to Health

Addressing the Root Cause

Herbalism seeks to identify and address the root cause of health issues rather than merely alleviating symptoms. It considers the person as a whole taking into account physical, emotional, and spiritual aspects.

Balancing Body Systems

Herbal remedies are often chosen to restore balance to the body's systems. Herbs are selected based on their specific actions whether it's supporting the digestive system, balancing hormones, or strengthening the immune system.

Mind-Body Connection

Holistic herbalism recognizes the intricate connection between mental and physical health. Herbs are chosen not only for their physiological effects but also for their impact on emotional well-being and mental clarity.

Nature as a Healing Partner

Respect for Nature's Wisdom

Herbalism acknowledges the wisdom inherent in nature. Plants are seen as teachers offering their healing properties to those who approach them with respect and understanding.

Ecosystem Health

The health of the ecosystem is considered in herbal practices. Sustainable harvesting, ethical wildcrafting, and promoting biodiversity are integral to maintaining the balance of the natural world.

Seasonal and Circadian Rhythms

Herbalism aligns with seasonal and circadian rhythms. The timing of harvesting, preparation, and administration of herbal remedies often takes into account the natural cycles of plants and the human body.

Preventative Care and Wellness

Nurturing Overall Well-Being

Herbalism emphasizes preventative care and overall wellness. Incorporating herbs into daily routines such as in teas, tonics, or culinary dishes supports the body in maintaining balance and resilience.

Strengthening the Body's Defenses

Herbs are used not only to treat specific ailments but also to strengthen the body's defenses, consequently enhancing its ability to resist illness and maintain optimal health.

Energy and Vitality

Vital Force and Energetics

Holistic herbalism considers the vital force or life energy present in plants. The energetics of herbs—whether warming or cooling —help match them to a person's constitution or specific health imbalances.

Adaptogens and Resilience

The use of adaptogenic herbs exemplifies the holistic approach. These herbs support the body's ability to adapt to stress, thus, promoting resilience and overall vitality.

Cultural and Spiritual Dimensions

Cultural Significance

Herbalism often holds cultural significance, integrating the cultural and spiritual dimensions of plant use. Plants are respected not only for their physical properties but also for their symbolism and role in cultural practices.

Spiritual Connection

Some herbal traditions incorporate spiritual practices, hence, recognize the spiritual connection between plants and humans. This may involve rituals, ceremonies, or mindfulness practices centered around herbal use.

Patient-Centered Care

Individualized Treatment

Holistic herbalism tailors treatments to the patient. A holistic herbalist considers the unique constitution, lifestyle, and emotional well-being of each person, recognizing that everyone is different.

Collaboration with Conventional Medicine

Holistic herbalism complements conventional medicine. Practitioners may work collaboratively with healthcare professionals to integrate herbal remedies into comprehensive healthcare plans.

Empowerment and Education

Empowering People

Herbalism empowers people to take an active role in their health. Through education and self-awareness, you can make informed choices about incorporating herbs into your lifestyle.

Community Education

Holistic herbalists often engage in educating the community, sharing knowledge about the benefits of herbal practices and, encouraging sustainable and mindful interactions with the natural world.

Closing Thoughts and Encouragement for the Budding Herbalist

As you embark on your herbal journey, take a moment to celebrate the curiosity and passion that led you here. Herbalism is a vast and enchanting world, filled with the wisdom of plants and the art of healing. Here are some friendly and detailed closing thoughts to inspire and support you along the green path.

Embrace the Learning Curve

Herbalism is a lifelong journey of discovery. Embrace the learning curve with an open heart and a gentle spirit. Every plant has a story to tell, and each lesson, whether easy or challenging, contributes to your growth as an herbalist.

Build a Relationship with Plants

Treat plants as your allies and friends. Get to know them intimately—observe, touch, smell, and listen. Building a relationship with plants goes beyond their medicinal properties; it is about understanding their spirit and the energy they bring.

Trust Your Intuition

In the world of herbs, intuition is a powerful guide. Listen to your inner wisdom as you choose herbs, create blends, and administer remedies. Your intuition—coupled with knowledge—will be a compass on your herbal journey.

Emphasize Sustainability

As stewards of the earth, practice sustainability in your herbalism. Learn ethical wildcrafting, support local growers, and strive to leave a positive footprint. The health of the planet is intricately connected to the health of the herbs you work with.

Connect with the Community

The herbal community is a source of inspiration and support. Connect with fellow herbalists, join workshops, attend conferences, or join online communities. Share your experiences, and maybe even inspire others to join the growing community of herbal enthusiasts worldwide. Together, we preserve the vibrant tapestry of humanity's herbal wisdom.

Be Patient with Your Progress

Rome was not built in a day and neither is herbal expertise. Be patient with your progress, celebrate small victories, and view challenges as opportunities for growth. Every step you take contributes to your becoming a more seasoned herbalist.

Document Your Herbal Experiences

Keep a journal of your herbal experiences. Note your observations, recipes, and the effects of different herbs. Your personal herbal journal will become a treasure trove of insights and memories along your herbal journey.

Continuously Learn and Stay Curious

Herbalism is a dynamic field with constant discoveries. Stay curious, read books, attend workshops, and stay abreast of the latest research. A curious mind is a fertile ground for an everblooming herbal practice.

Celebrate Nature's Cycles

Align your herbal practices with the cycles of nature. Observe the changing seasons, lunar phases, and the ebb and flow of plant life. Nature is the ultimate teacher, and attuning yourself to its rhythms enhances your herbal wisdom.

Trust in the Healing Process

Healing is a holistic journey that involves the body, mind, and spirit. Trust in the healing process—both for yourself and those you may guide. Herbs work in harmony with the body's innate wisdom, promoting holistic well-being.

Closing Note

We at The Green Glow sincerely hope this journey into the world of herbs has been enlightening and empowering for you. Continue your learning journey by joining the passionate group of herbal enthusiasts at *Herbs, Hearts, and Healing* on Facebook! Participate in discussions on herbal remedies, share knowledge, or seek advice at www. facebook. com/ groups/ 632684879060409.

Your understanding of the incredible potential of herbal remedies is now just beginning to sprout. Remember, you are joining a lineage of healers who have revered and worked with plants for centuries. As you venture into the magical realm of herbalism, know that you are contributing to a legacy of natural healing and harmony.

If you enjoyed learning about herbs, history, holistic health, and horticulture, please share your thoughts and experiences through a review. Your feedback is invaluable and can help others discover the transformative benefits of herbalism.

Thank you for joining us on this herbal adventure, and may your path be filled with health, harmony, and a deep connection to our natural world that comes from cultivating a green path.

Green blessings on your herbal adventure!

Thanks For Reading!

Hey! Thanks for taking the time to read this and may the seeds of knowledge we've planted grow and flourish. One last thing, and at this point we probably sound like a broken record, but it would mean a great deal to us if you left a review. Also, don't forget to grab your freebie if you haven't already! Just scan the code. See you in the Facebook group!

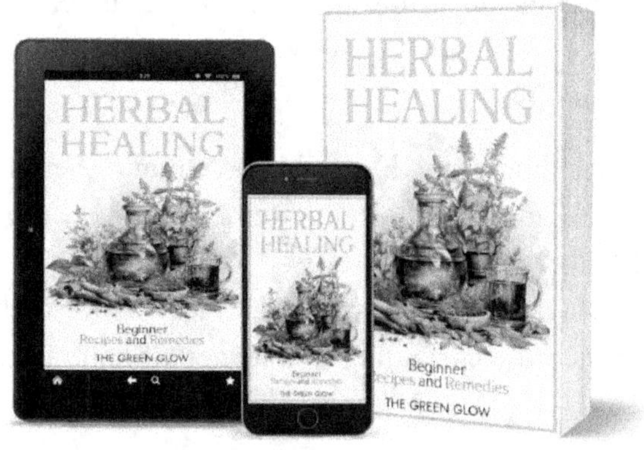

Yes, I almost forgot my freebie

Adeleye, O. A., Femi-Oyewo, M. N., Bamiro, O. A., Bakre, L. G., Alabi, A., Ashidi, J. S., Balogun-Agbaje, O. A., Hassan, O. M., & Fakoya, G. (2021). Ethnomedicinal herbs in african traditional medicine with potential activity for the prevention, treatment, and management of coronavirus disease 2019. *Future Journal of Pharmaceutical Sciences*, 7(1). https:// doi.org/ 10.1186/ s43094-021-00223-5

Seven medicinal health benefits of strophanthus courmontii (climbing oleander). (2023a, August 27). Agric4Profits. https:/ / agric4profits.com/ 7-medicinal-health-benefits-of-strophanthus-courmontii-climbing-oleander/

Twelve *medicinal health benefits of alangium chinense (chinese alangium)*. (2. 023b, August 30)Agric4profits. https:/ / agric4profits.com/ 12-medicinal-health-benefits-of-alangium-chinense-chinese-alangium/

Ajmera, R. (2017). *Eight benefits of hibiscus tea*. Healthline. https:/ / www.healthline.com/ nutrition/ hibiscus-tea-benefits

Ajmera, R., & Hill, A. (2018). *Thirteen potential health benefits of dandelion*. Healthline. https:/ / www.healthline.com/ nutrition/ dandelion-benefits

Tatarian aster root (aster tataricus). (2023). All Things Health. https:/ / www.allthingshealth.com/ en-my/ glossary/ tatarian-aster-root-aster-tataricus/

Ally. (2023a, January 2). *Parsley companion plants*. Boreal Bloom Homestead. https:/ / borealbloomhomestead.com/ parsley-companion-plants/

Ally. (2023b, January 3). D*ill companion plants {and some to avoid}*. Boreal Bloom Homestead. https:/ / borealbloomhomestead.com/ dill-companion-plants/

Ally. (2023c, January 7). *Sage companion plants*. Boreal Bloom Homestead. https:/ / borealbloomhomestead.com/ sage-companion-plants/

Aloi, P. (2021, June 25). *How to grow and care for valerian*. The Spruce. https:/ / www.thespruce.com/ how-to-grow-valerian-5088230

Aremu, A. O., & Makunga, N. (2022, July 12). *Africa is a treasure trove of medicinal plants: Here are seven that are popular*. The Conversation. https:/ / theconversation.com/ africa-is-a-treasure-trove-of-medicinal-plants-here-are-seven-that-are-popular-184189

Arnarson, A. (2018, May 4). *Six science-based health benefits of moringa oleifera*. Healthline. https:/ / www.healthline.com/ nutrition/ 6-benefits-of-moringa-oleifera

Bibliography

Chitrak: Getting to know your herbal allies. (2017a, January 20). Banyan Botanicals. https:/ / www.banyanbotanicals.com/ info/ blog-the-banyan-insight/ details/ getting-to-know-your-herbal-allies-chitrak/

. *Shardunika (gymnema sylvestre): Getting to know your herbal allies.* (2017b, March 15). Banyan Botanicals. https:/ / www.banyanbotanicals.com/ info/ blog-the-banyan-insight/ details/ getting-to-know-your-herbal-allies-shardunika/

. *Ginger: Getting to know your herbal allies.* (2017c, April 7). Banyan Botanicals. https:/ / www.banyanbotanicals.com/ info/ blog-the-banyan-insight/ details/ getting-to-know-your-herbal-allies-ginger/

. *Manjistha: Getting to know your herbal allies.* Banyan Botanicals. https:/ / www.banyanbotanicals.com/ info/ blog-the-banyan-insight/ details/ getting-to-know-your-herbal-allies-manjistha/

Brahmi/ Gotu kola: Getting to know your herbal allies. (2017e, August 17).Banyan Botanicals. https:/ / www.banyanbotanicals.com/ info/ blog-the-banyan-insight/ details/ getting-to-know-your-herbal-allies-brahmi-gotu-kola-centella-asiatica/

Banyan Botanicals. (2017f, December 14). *Kalmegh: Getting to know your herbal allies.* Banyan Botanicals. https:/ / www.banyanbotanicals.com/ info/ blog-the-banyan-insight/ details/ getting-to-know-your-herbal-allies-kalmegh/

Licorice: Getting to know your herbal allies. (2018, March 12). Banyan Botanicals. https:/ / www.banyanbotanicals.com/ info/ blog-the-banyan-insight/ details/ herbal-allies-licorice-glycyrrhiza-glabra/

Pippali: Getting to know your herbal allies. (2019a, January 15). Banyan Botanicals. https:/ / www.banyanbotanicals.com/ info/ blog-the-banyan-insight/ details/ getting-to-know-your-herbal-allies-pippali-piper-longum/

Fennel: Getting to know your herbal allies. (2019b, April 10). Banyan Botanicals. https:/ / www.banyanbotanicals.com/ info/ blog-the-banyan-insight/ details/ fennel-foeniculum-vulgare/

Vasaka: Getting to know your herbal allies. (2020, May 26). Banyan Botanicals. https:/ / www.banyanbotanicals.com/ info/ blog-the-banyan-insight/ details/ getting-to-know-your-herbal-allies-vasaka/

Ayurvedic herbs. (2024). Banyan Botanicals. https:/ / www.banyanbotanicals.-com/ info/ plants/ ayurvedic-herbs/

Basu, S. (2023, November 16). *Dill leaves: Astonishing benefits of adding this nutritious herb to your diet.* Netmeds. https:/ / www.netmeds.com/ health-library/ post/ dill-leaves-astonishing-benefits-of-adding-this-nutritious-herb-to-your-diet

Bennett, C. (2019, November 26). *The health benefits of cilantro (coriander).*

News-Medical Life Sciences. https:/ / www.news-medical.net/ health/ The-Health-Benefits-of-Cilantro-(Coriander).aspx

Berkheiser, K. (2020, August 12). *Guggul: Benefits, dosage, side effects, and more*. Healthline. https:/ / www.healthline.com/ nutrition/ guggul

Ten *rosemary companion plants (& 5 plants to keep far away)*. (2021, November 11). Blooming Backyard. https:/ / www.bloomingbackyard.com/ rosemary-companion-plants/

Boeckmann, C. (2023a, November). *Japanese beetles*. Old Farmer's Almanac. https:/ / www.almanac.com/ pest/ japanese-beetles

Boeckmann, C. (2023b, November 21). *Herb planting calendar: Planting and growing herbs*. Old Farmer's Almanac. https:/ / www.almanac.com/ herb-growing-guide-how-grow-herbs

Boness, K. (2023, January 18). *StackPath*. Gardeningknowhow. https:/ / www.-gardeningknowhow.com/ edible/ herbs/ borage/ companion-planting-with-borage.htm

How to grow chives | quick guide to growing chives. (2023). Bonnie Plants. https:/ / bonnieplants.com/ blogs/ how-to-grow/ growing-chives

Caliskaner, Z., Kartal, O., Gulec, M., Ozturk, S., Erel, F., Sener, O., & Karaayvaz, M. (2010). Awareness of allergy patients about herbal remedies: A cross-sectional study of residents of ankara, turkey. *Allergologia et Immunopathologia*, *38*(2), 78–82. https:/ / doi.org/ 10.1016/ j.aller.2009.07.010

Cazzola, R., & Cestaro, B. (2014, January 1). *Chapter 9-antioxidant spices and herbs used in diabetes*. ScienceDirect; Academic Press. https:/ / www.sci-encedirect.com/ science/ article/ abs/ pii/ B9780124058859000097

Chappell, S. (2019, February 21). *A beginner's guide to making herbal salves and lotions*. Healthline. https:/ / www.healthline.com/ health/ diy-herbal-salves#rash-cream-recipe

Cheryl M. (2021, September 4). *Fifty herbs and spices from a-z*. Everyday Family Favorites. https:/ / everydayfamilyfavorites.wordpress.com/ author/ everydayfamilyfavorites/

Clark, C. (2022, September 8). *Herbalist tools-get started with herbalism*. Zyto. https:/ / zyto.com/ 17-best-herbalist-tools

Cronkleton, E. (2017, September 19). *Gotu kola: 10 benefits, side effects, and more*. Healthline. https:/ / www.healthline.com/ health/ gotu-kola-bene-fits#wound-healing-and-scarring

Danahy, A. (2021, July 9). *What is giloy? Nutrients, benefits, downsides, and more*. Healthline. https:/ / www.healthline.com/ nutrition/ giloy-benefits

DaSilva, Z. S. (2017). *The herb in history, mysteries and crafts*. https:/ / www.-cambridgescholars.com/ resources/ pdfs/ 978-1-4438-5687-4-sample.pdf

Bibliography

Dharmananda, S. (2023). *Major European herbs - chapter 2: Tracing the history of European herbology.* ITM Online. http:/ / www.itmonline.org/ kunzle/ chap2.htm

DiSanti, J. (2019, July 23). *Homemade coconut vanilla cardamom granola.* Mountain Rose Herbs. https:/ / blog.mountainroseherbs.com/ coconut-cardamom-granola

Duke, J. A. (2013). *Handbook of medicinal herbs.* Crc Press.

Dylan. (2023a, April 14). *Nine best cilantro companion plants (+ 11 to avoid).* Make It Seasonal. https:/ / makeitseasonal.com/ cilantro-companion-planting/

Dylan. (2023b, April 20). *Twelve basil companion plants for a healthier garden.* Make It Seasonal. https:/ / makeitseasonal.com/ basil-companion-plants/

Dylan. (2023c, April 20). *Thirteen best mint companion plants for a healthier garden.* Make It Seasonal. https:/ / makeitseasonal.com/ mint-companion-plants/

Dylan. (2023d, April 30). *Twelve best chives companion plants for a better harvest.* Make It Seasonal. https:/ / makeitseasonal.com/ chives-companion-plants/ #the-best-companion-plants-for-chives

Dylan. (2023e, May 12). *Eight best thyme companion plants (+ 8 to avoid).* Make It Seasonal. https:/ / makeitseasonal.com/ thyme-companion-plants/

Dylan. (2023f, May 24). *The 11 best companion plants for oregano.* Make It Seasonal. https:/ / makeitseasonal.com/ oregano-companion-plants/

Ersek, K. (2011). *The science behind holganix: Monocots vs dicots: What you need to know.* Holganix. https:/ / www.holganix.com/ blog/ monocots-vs-dicots-what-you-need-to-know

Fanous, S. (2014, November 4). *Nine health benefits of thyme.* Healthline. https:/ / www.healthline.com/ health/ health-benefits-of-thyme

Fawn, S. (2020, April 3). *Magical herbal medicine of the ancient egyptians.* Iseum Sanctuary. https:/ / iseumsanctuary.com/ 2020/ 04/ 02/ magical-herbal-medicine-of-the-ancient-egyptians/

Ferment, G. F. C. (2020, December 6). *Fiveteen best books on herbalism and natural body care.* Grow Forage Cook Ferment. https:/ / www.growforage-cookferment.com/ herbalism-books/

Firdous, H. (2024). *Manjishtha (rubia cordifolia) benefits and its side effects.* Lybrate. https:/ / www.lybrate.com/ topic/ manjishtha-rubia-cordifolia-benefits-and-side-effects

Foster, S. (2023). *A brief history of adulteration of herbs, spices, and botanical drugs-american botanical council.* Herbalgram. https:/ / www.herbalgram.org/ resources/ herbalgram/ issues/ 92/ table-of-contents/ feat-hxadulteration/

Fotolio LLC. (2011). *Bitterroot (Lakota name: Sinkpe tawote. Scientific name: Acorus calamus), 2011.* Native Voices. https:/ / www.nlm.nih.gov/ nativevoices/ exhibition/ healing-ways/ medicine-ways/ healing-plants/ images/ ob1680.html

Francis, M. (2024). *Healing herbs: Learn to make infused oils and balms.* HGTV. https:/ / www.hgtv.com/ design/ make-and-celebrate/ handmade/ healing-herbs-learn-to-make-infused-oils-and-balms

Gallagher, G. (2019, October 25). *Bhringraj oil health benefits, uses, side effects, and precautions.* Healthline. https:/ / www.healthline.com/ health/ bhringraj-oil#What-is-bhringraj-oil?

Galper, A. (2022, January 18). *Carrier oils vs essential oils - what's the difference!?* Cliganic. https:/ / www.cliganic.com/ blogs/ the-essentials/ carrier-oils-vs-essential-oils

Gardenia. (2024). *Echinacea purpurea (purple coneflower).* Gardenia.net. https:/ / www.gardenia.net/ plant/ echinacea-purpurea

Gardiner, B. (2021, February 14). *Nine basic principles of ethical wildcrafting for beginners.* The Outdoor Apothecary. https:/ / www.outdoorapothecary.-com/ ethical-wildcrafting

Gianni, K. (2018, May 20). *A beginner's 5-step guide to wildcrafting.* Annmarie Skin Care. https:/ / www.annmariegianni.com/ beginners-guide-ethical-wildcrafting/

Goldman, R. (2014, December 4). *Comfrey: Uses, risks, and takeaways.* Healthline. https:/ / www.healthline.com/ health/ what-is-comfrey#uses

Goodson, A. (2018, June 18). *Six impressive health benefits of gymnema sylvestre.* Healthline; Healthline Media. https:/ / www.healthline.com/ nutri-tion/ gymnema-sylvestre-benefits

Green Glow Gatherings. (2023). *Herbs, hearts, and healing.* Facebook. https:/ / www.facebook.com/ groups/ 632684879060409

Greenfield, O. (2023, May 3). *Thirty-three best bee balm companion plants.* Balcony Garden Web. https:/ / balconygardenweb.com/ bee-balm-compan-ion-plants/

Hannan, J. (2023, February). *How to change your soil's pH.* Iowa State University Extension and Outreach. https:/ / hortnews.extension.iastate.edu/ how-change-your-soils-ph

Hellicar, L. (2022, November 15). *Tarragon health benefits: Skin, hair, diges-tion, and more.* Medical News Today. https:/ / www.medicalnewstoday.-com/ articles/ tarragon-benefits

Herbal Africa. (2021). Natural plants used in our product range. In *Herbal Africa.* https:/ / herbalafrica.co.za/ wp-content/ uploads/ 2021/ 09/ South-African-Medicinal-Plants-Manual.pdf

Bibliography

Heron, B. (2023, January 25). *How to make a herbal salve.* Earthsong Seeds. https:/ / earthsongseeds.co.uk/ recipes/ how-to-make-a-herbal-salve/

Hill, A. (2019, December 6). *Caraway: nutrients, benefits, and uses.* Healthline. https:/ / www.healthline.com/ nutrition/ caraway

Hopkins, M. (2013, April 1). *The role of gypsum in agriculture: 5 key benefits you should know.* CropLife. https:/ / www.croplife.com/ crop-inputs/ micronutrients/ the-role-of-gypsum-in-agriculture-5-key-benefits-you-should-know/

Hu, X.-Y., Wei, X., Zhou, Y.-Q., Liu, X.-W., Li, J.-X., Zhang, W., Wang, C.-B., Zhang, L.-Y., & Zhou, Y. (2020, November 1). *Genus Alangium-A review on its traditional uses, phytochemistry and pharmacological activities.* Fitoterapia. https:/ / doi.org/ 10.1016/ j.fitote.2020.104773

Hunter, C. (2008, October 17). *How to make an herbal oil: cold infused botanical oils.* The Practical Herbalist. https:/ / thepracticalherbalist.com/ advanced-herbalism/ making-a-cold-infused-herbal-oil-a-general-procedure/

Iannotti, M. (2023, March 20). *How to grow thyme.* The Spruce. https:/ / www.thespruce.com/ how-to-grow-thyme-1402630

Irene. (2017, June 13). *How to make herbal salves.* Mountain Rose Herbs. https:/ / blog.mountainroseherbs.com/ diy-herbal-salves

Izuchukwu, O. J. (2024). *The history of African traditional medicine.* Academia. https:/ / www.academia.edu/ 36040250/ THE_HISTORY_OF_AFRICAN_TRADITIONAL_MEDICINE

Jabbour, N. (2021, June 18). *How to harvest herbs: how and when to harvest homegrown herbs.* Savvy Gardening. https:/ / savvygardening.com/ how-to-harvest-herbs/

Jarić, S., Kostić, O., Mataruga, Z., Pavlović, D., Pavlović, M., Mitrović, M., & Pavlović, P. (2018). Traditional wound-healing plants used in the Balkan region (Southeast Europe). *Journal of Ethnopharmacology, 211*(211), 311–328. https:/ / doi.org/ 10.1016/ j.jep.2017.09.018

Jennings, M. (2014, November 2). *PPT-A global overview of herbal/ traditional products powerpoint presentation - ID:6082660.* SlideServe. https:/ / www.slideserve.com/ melyssa-jennings/ a-global-overview-of-herbal-traditional-products

Jess. (2017, September 22). *Balms vs. salves: Is there really a difference?* Pronounce Skincare & Herbal Boutique. https:/ / pronounceskincare.com/ balms-vs-salves-is-there-a-difference/

Jones, S. (2018, April 7). *Companion planting dandelions (no...really!).* Growing Guides. https:/ / growing-guides.co.uk/ companion-planting-dandelions/

Karadsheh, S. (2022, April 21). *Best way to store fresh herbs (2 easy methods).*

The Mediterranean Dish. https:/ / www.themediterraneandish.com/ how-to-store-fresh-herbs/

Kolen, R. (2017, June 13). *How to make herbal tinctures.* Mountain Rose Herbs. https:/ / blog.mountainroseherbs.com/ guide-tinctures-extracts

Kolen, R. (2018, May 21). *How to make your own herbal capsules.* Mountainroseherbs. https:/ / blog.mountainroseherbs.com/ diy-herbal-capsules

Krans, B. (2014, October 13). *The health benefits of holy basil.* Healthline; Healthline Media. https:/ / www.healthline.com/ health/ food-nutrition/ basil-benefits

Kubala, J. (2021, October 18). *Five potential health benefits of lemon verbena.* Healthline. https:/ / www.healthline.com/ nutrition/ lemon-verbena-uses

Lang, A. (2021, January 20). *Camellia sinensis leaf extract: Benefits, uses, and side effects.* Healthline. https:/ / www.healthline.com/ nutrition/ camellia-sinensis-leaf-extract

Laura. (2020, April 24). *Dandelion cream scones.* Lonely Pines Farm. https:/ / www.lonelypinesfarm.com/ dandelion-cream-scones/

Leech, J. (2020, May 15). *Aloe vera: 8 health benefits.* Medical News Today. https:/ / www.medicalnewstoday.com/ articles/ 318591#dental-plaque

Lin, N. (2017). *Korean mint–roots of medicine.* Roots of Medicine. https:/ / dsps.lib.uiowa.edu/ roots/ korean-mint

Magyar, C. (2022, March 16). *Fourteen lesser-known herbs that deserve a spot in your herb garden.* Rural Sprout. https:/ / www.ruralsprout.com/ lesser-known-herbs/

Map Expo. (2017, May 26). *Twenty-three medicinal plants the Native Americans used on a daily basis.* MAP-Expo. https:/ / map-expo.com/ high-lights/ 23-medicinal-plants-native-americans-used-daily-basis/

Marceau , H. (2014, October 20). *The importance of plant identification–part 1.* Phyto Chemia. https:/ / phytochemia.com/ en/ 2014/ 10/ 20/ the-impor-tance-of-plant-identification-part-1/

Marie, J. (2024). *Herb leaf identification.* Ehow. https:/ / www.ehow.com/ fact-s_7664931_herb-leaf-identification.html

McDermott, A. (2017, October 10). *Shatavari: benefits, side effects, and more.* Healthline. https:/ / www.healthline.com/ health/ food-nutrition/ shatavari

McGruther, J. (2023a, March 23). *Swap lettuce for fresh herbs in your salad. you'll thank me later.* Nourished Kitchen. https:/ / nourishedkitchen.com/ herb-salad/

McGruther, J. (2023b, November 12). *Want to make the best gingerbread? It starts with this ancient grain.* Nourished Kitchen. https:/ / nourished-kitchen.com/ einkorn-gingerbread/

McGruther, J. (2023c, December 28). *How to make caraway sauerkraut (great for gut health!).* Nourished Kitchen. https:/ / nourishedkitchen.com/ caraway-sauerkraut/

McLaughlin, C. (2010, June 14). *The benefits of raised garden beds.* FineGardening. https:/ / www.finegardening.com/ article/ the-benefits-of-raised-garden-beds

McMullan, C. (2020, October 19). *Mint growing and harvest information.* VeggieHarvest. https:/ / veggieharvest.com/ herbs/ mint-growing-and-harvest-information/

Moncivaiz, A. (2013, October 23). *Boswellia: Uses, dosage, side effects, and more.* Healthline. https:/ / www.healthline.com/ health/ boswellia#side-effects

Comfrey information. (2024a). Mount Sinai Health System. https:/ / www.-mountsinai.org/ health-library/ herb/ comfrey

Echinacea information. (2024b). Mount Sinai Health System. https:/ / www.-mountsinai.org/ health-library/ herb/ echinacea

Plant information: Safflower. (2024). Mountain Herb Estate. https:/ / www.herbgarden.co.za/ mountainherb/ herbinfo.php?id=516

Murray, D. (2023). *Can fennel increase your breast milk supply and is it safe?* Verywell Family. https:/ / www.verywellfamily.com/ fennel-breastfeeding-and-increasing-breast-milk-supply-431838

Traditional Chinese medicine: What you need to know. (2019, April). NCCIH. https:/ / www.nccih.nih.gov/ health/ traditional-chinese-medicine-what-you-need-to-know

Dietary and herbal supplements. (2020). NCCIH. https:/ / www.nccih.nih.gov/ health/ dietary-and-herbal-supplements

Valerian. (2020, October). NCCIH. https:/ / www.nccih.nih.gov/ health/ valerian

Herb-drug Interactions. (2021, July). NCCIH. https:/ / www.nccih.nih.gov/ health/ providers/ digest/ herb-drug-interactions

Ortega, P. (2011). *Paul Ortega with large Yucca plant, Mescalero, New Mexico, 2011.* Native Voices. https:/ / www.nlm.nih.gov/ nativevoices/ exhibition/ healing-ways/ medicine-ways/ healing-plants/ images/ ob1676.html

Ozioma, E.-O. J., & Nwamaka Chinwe, O. A. (2019, January 30). *Herbal medicines in african traditional medicine.* IntechOpen. https:/ / www.intechopen.com/ chapters/ 64851

Pacheco, E. (2023, April 25). *Companion planting with stinging nettle: The best plants to grow together.* Shuncy. https:/ / shuncy.com/ article/ what-are-the-best-companion-plants-for-stinging-nettle

Parmar, R. (2022, April 7). *11 incredible health benefits of fennel seeds (saunf).* PharmEasy Blog. https:/ / pharmeasy.in/ blog/ 10-incredible-health-benefits-of-fennel-seeds-saunf/

Partnership for Environmental Education and Rural Health. (2024). Partnership for environmental education and rural health medicinal plants of the american indians. In *Texas A&M School of Veterinary Medicine & Biomedical Sciences*. https:/ / vetmed.tamu.edu/ peer/ wp-content/ uploads/ sites/ 72/ 2020/ 04/ DLC808_Medicinal-Plants-of-North-America.pdf

PCC Institute for Health Professionals. (2021, February 20). What herbalism is and why it's important today. *Portland Community College*. https:/ / climb.pcc.edu/ blog/ what-herbalism-is-and-why-its-important-today

Pitman, V. (2017, December 7). *Ancient medicine, herbs and herbal practice*. Herbal History Research Network. https:/ / www.herbalhistory.org/ home/ ancient-medicine-herbs-and-herbal-practice/

Planet Natural. (2023). *How to get rid of thrips*. Planet Natural. https:/ / www.-planetnatural.com/ pest-problem-solver/ houseplant-pests/ thrips-control/

Pole, S. (2023, January 24). *How to make an infused massage oil*. Earthsong Seeds. https:/ / earthsongseeds.co.uk/ recipes/ how-to-make-an-infused-massage-oil/

Pulikkotti, A. J. (2018). *Medicinal plants of india ; ayurveda*. Indian Medicinal Plants. https:/ / indianmedicinalplants.info/ index.htm

Raman, R. (2019, October 31). *7 emerging benefits of bacopa monnieri (brahmi)*. Healthline. https:/ / www.healthline.com/ nutrition/ bacopa-monnieri-benefits#TOC_TITLE_HDR_4

Raye, J. (2019, May 8). *5 steps to take herbal medicine safely*. Jennifer Raye Medicine and Movement. https:/ / jenniferraye.com/ herbal-safety/

Regina. (2022, January 12). *Planting fennel: Seeds, companion plants & more*. Plantura. https:/ / plantura.garden/ uk/ vegetables/ fennel/ planting-fennel

Richins, R. D. (2011a). *Mescal plant, New Mexico, 2011*. Native Voices. https:/ / www.nlm.nih.gov/ nativevoices/ exhibition/ healing-ways/ medicine-ways/ healing-plants/ images/ ob1677.html

Richins, R. D. (2011b). *Mesquite plant, New Mexico, 2011*. Native Voices. https:/ / www.nlm.nih.gov/ nativevoices/ exhibition/ healing-ways/ medicine-ways/ healing-plants/ images/ ob1678.html

Robinson, K. (2021). *Differences between conventional medicine and homeopathy*. Homeopathy Yes. https:/ / homeopathyyes.com/ case-studies/ principles-and-practice-of/ differences-between-convent.html

Ruggeri, C. (2018, July 22). *The top 101 herbs and spices for healing*. Dr. Axe. https:/ / draxe.com/ nutrition/ top-herbs-spices-healing/

Sara. (2017, June 28). *Paleo ashwagandha chocolate bites*. Mountain Rose Herbs. https:/ / blog.mountainroseherbs.com/ paleo-ashwagandha-chocolate-bites

Schneider, A. (2011). *Osha (Lakota name: Mato tapejuta. Scientific name: Ligusticum porter) - Healing Plants - Medicine Ways: Traditional Healers and Healing - Healing Ways - Exhibition - Native Voices*. Native Voices. https:/ / www.nlm.nih.gov/ nativevoices/ exhibition/ healing-ways/ medicine-ways/ healing-plants/ images/ ob1681.html

Seegers, B. (2018, October 2). *Featured plant: Jindai tatarian aster*. The High Line. https:/ / www.thehighline.org/ blog/ 2018/ 10/ 02/ featured-plant-jindai-tartarian-aster/

Semb, H. (2023, April 25). *Tips for growing dandelions with companion plants*. Shuncy. https:/ / shuncy.com/ article/ what-companion-plants-grow-well-with-dandelions

Sencha Tea Bar. (2024). *Tea for beginners: The ultimate guide to tea basics*. Sencha Tea Bar. https:/ / senchateabar.com/ blogs/ blog/ tea-for-beginners

Sheff, E. (2015, November 3). *Making herbal pills*. Linkedin. https:/ / www.linkedin.com/ pulse/ making-herbal-pills-elaine-sheff

Sherwood, D. (2023, June 6). *9 tips for growing thyme in pots or containers*. Epic Gardening. https:/ / www.epicgardening.com/ thyme-containers/

Singh, R. (2022, March 9). *Pippali: Uses, benefits, side effects & more!* PharmEasy Blog. https:/ / pharmeasy.in/ blog/ ayurveda-uses-benefits-side-effects-of-pippali/

Singh, R. (2023, February 19). *Vasaka: Uses, benefits and side effects by dr. rajeev singh*. PharmEasy Blog. https:/ / pharmeasy.in/ blog/ ayurveda-uses-benefits-and-side-effects-of-vasaka

Sobel, A. (2019, July 18). *10 science-backed benefits of sesame oil*. Healthline. https:/ / www.healthline.com/ nutrition/ sesame-oil-benefits#TOC_TITLE_HDR_7

South African Fynbos. (2024). *Rhino Bush*. South African Fynbos. https:/ / www.southafricanfynbos.com/ collections/ rhino-bush

Sruthi, M. (2022, October 8). *8 health benefits of lemon verbena: Uses, side effects, tea*. MedicineNet. https:/ / www.medicinenet.com/ 8_health_benefits_of_lemon_verbena/ article.htm

St.Amant, K. (2019, August 8). *Contextualizing care in cultures: Perspectives on cross-cultural and international health and medical communication – present tense*. Present Tense Journal. http:/ / www.presenttensejournal.org/ editorial/ contextualizing-care-in-cultures-perspectives-on-cross-cultural-and-international-health-and-medical-communication/

Strassburg, N. (2024). *Herb companion plants*. Nathalie Strassburg. https:/ / nathaliestrassburg.com/ the-medicine-garden/ herb-companion-plants/

Teall, E. K. (2014). Medicine and doctoring in ancient Mesopotamia. *Grand Valley Journal of History*, 3(1). https:/ / scholarworks.gvsu.edu/ cgi/ viewcontent.cgi?article=1056&context=gvjh

Thiele, J. (2023, April 4). *How to make a herbal tincture*. Herbal Reality.

https:/ / www.herbalreality.com/ herbalism/ home-herbalism/ making-medicines/ how-to-make-herbal-tincture

Tieraona Low Dog. (2021, August 25). *How to make elderberry syrup for immune system support.* Mountain Rose Herbs. https:/ / blog.mountainroseherbs.com/ elderberry-syrup-recipe

Toshi, N. (2020, August 17). *Twelve health benefits of mint leaves that you should know!* PharmEasy Blog. https:/ / pharmeasy.in/ blog/ benefits-of-mint-leaves/

Turley, D. (2017, March 22). *Don't guess — know these popular herbal supplement doses.* Charlottes Book. https:/ / www.charlottesbook.com/ herbal-supplement-doses/

Urban Moonshine. (2024). *Three ways to tap into an herbal community near you.* Urban Moonshine. https:/ / www.urbanmoonshine.com/ blogs/ blog/ 3-ways-to-tap-into-an-herbal-community-near-you

USDA. (2023). *Medicinal botany.* U.S. Forest Service. https:/ / www.fs.usda.gov/ wildflowers/ ethnobotany/ medicinal/

van Zon, P. (2018, March 20). *Do you see the difference between real and artificial?* Bloomifique. https:/ / bloomifique.com/ en/ see-difference-real-artificial/

Traditional chinese medicine-A brief history. (2020, October). Village Remedies. https:/ / www.villageremedies.com/ blog-articles/ traditional-chinese-medicine-a-brief-history

Visser, M. (2015, February 11). *Determining herbal dosages.* Growing up Herbal. https:/ / growingupherbal.com/ herbal-dosages/

Wagner, C., De Gezelle, J., & Komarnytsky, S. (2020). Celtic provenance in traditional herbal medicine of medieval Wales and classical antiquity. *Frontiers in Pharmacology, 11*(105). https:/ / doi.org/ 10.3389/ fphar.2020.00105

Watson, K. (2018, December 5). *Aloe vera for psoriasis: Benefits, uses, and more.* Healthline. https:/ / www.healthline.com/ health/ aloe-vera-for-psoriasis#1

West, H. (2018, January 19). *Seven science-based benefits of milk thistle.* Healthline; Healthline Media. https:/ / www.healthline.com/ nutrition/ milk-thistle-benefits

Wynn, F. (2019, February 19). *What is energetic herbalism?* The Thirlby. https:/ / www.thethirlby.com/ thejournal/ 2019/ 2/ 19/ what-is-energetic-herbalism

Yoder, S. (2023, July 12). *Seven caraway companion plants & 4 to avoid.* Garden Housing. https:/ / garden-housing.com/ gardening/ 7-caraway-companion-plants-4-to-avoid/

Ziton, T. (2022, October 18). *The top 10 companion plants for echinacea (coneflower)*. Couch to Homestead. https:/ / couchtohomestead.com/ cone-flower-companion-plants/

Ziton, T. (2023, February 5). *Companion planting comfrey (benefits, pairings, & more)*. Couch to Homestead. https:/ / couchtohomestead.com/ comfrey-companion-plants/

9 798886 399229